REBEL DIET

Trade mark number: 2484721

REBEL DIET

Emma James
MABNLP, MATLTA, MABH, Dip FTST, IHHTT

First edition
Published in Great Britain
By Mirage Publishing 2008

Text Copyright © Emma James 2008

First published in paperback 2008

No part of this publication may be reproduced,
stored in a retrieval system or transmitted in any
form or by any means without first seeking
the written authority from the publisher.
The purchase or possession of this book
in any form deems acceptance
of these conditions.

A CIP catalogue record for this book
Is available from the British Library.

ISBN: 978-1-90257-838-5

Mirage Publishing
PO Box 161
Gateshead
NE8 4WW
Great Britain

www.miragepublishing.com

Printed and bound in Great Britain by

Book Printing UK
Remus House, Coltsfoot Drive, Woodston, Peterborough, PE2 9JX

Cover © Mirage Publishing
Layout by Artistic Director Sharon Anderson

Papers used in the production of this book are recycled,
thus reducing environmental depletion.

Dedicated to my Father, William Victor James
MRCS (Eng) LRCP (Lond) MBBS (Lond) FRCS (Ed)
(4th April 1923 to 15th January 2008)

My inspiration, irritator, friend and strength
You taught me belief, justice and the right to being individual

I know you are with me always

Contents

    Preface   ix

1. They don't want you to have it! Why?   11
2. The Diet Industry   19
3. Understanding You & The Stress Monsters   27
4. Your Motivation (or lack of it)   37
5. Self Esteem, Mistakes and Faux pas   45
6. Body Image & The 3 Me's   51
7. Metabolic Monster   59
8. The Knicker Effect   67
9. Fast & Slow Metabolic Rates   73
10. Nutrition   79
11. What rebels are not told   85
12. The diets & when to use them   91
13. So, give me the bad news. What *can* I eat?   97
14. The nitty gritty!   105
15. Confuse that Nemesis!   125
16. Exercise   131
17. Sympathetic Supplements   145
18. Where do I go from here then?   153

Troubleshooting Rebel   155
Other Titles   161

Preface

'The ability to change is borne from learning excellence. To bend to the winds which blow and might break you, creates new unique branches which will one day become the root of the new generation.'

Emma James

My life has been a myriad of amazing people, life experiences, training, competing and the welding together of all those things into the Training and Therapy business I have today.

Without the personal traumas, tribulations and 'terribles' that I have experienced throughout life, I wouldn't have gained the information necessary to write this book and my life would never have taken the course it has.

The book you are holding is the culmination of work, research, life lessons and the many wonderful clients who have amazed me with their spirit and determination to overcome the most crushing incidents which would have stopped many of us in our tracks.

It also emanates from the loathing of red tape and bureaucracy which intertwines itself through our lives like creeping vines, disguised as comfort when in fact it is eating away at our very foundations.

My belief and career has been emblazoned with the conviction that we are all individual and, as such, no one therapy, diet, strategy or lifestyle will fit all of us. I also believe that with such mass media, marketing and misinformation, our trust has been betrayed in the areas which we hold important, like our own self image and esteem. As a result, those who have a bit of a slow metabolism for various reasons then become the prey, and the key information you need is never quite given, keeping you coming back for more.

The information in here is designed to set you free

It is there to give you the insight into your mental state and the effect it will have on your success in getting to and maintaining the weight you want and the look you want. It will also turn around your attitude and belief in yourself and your ability in all the other areas of your life you want to succeed in.

It will show you the link between your mental state and your body and how the performance of one will affect the other, how to change it and what you are dealing with.

It also shows you how to get to know your body, your metabolism and know what to do and when to achieve the look you want.

This book is intended to be the last one you buy in the 'diet' section, to give you the information you need for life and therefore give the power back to *you* instead of the diet industry.

As a result of the success achieved by so many clients who used my approach, I was told to write a book, instead of breathing fire and brimstone about the 'mystery' being built up around diet and disempowering messages that only other people can do it for you.

Those who know me well know my own battle with weight while, those who don't, assume that because I compete and because of the way I look, I never had that battle. The endless 'gurus' who couldn't understand why I wasn't losing body fat with the level of training and diet I was on just pushed me into finding my own answers, which then proved to be the answers that thousands of others were looking for.

From my career as an NLP & Hypnosis Trainer and Master Practitioner Therapist, specialising in eating and weight related disorders, I knew the connection between emotional state and metabolism. I therefore began to put together research and notes about the findings and effectiveness of addressing these issues within a weight management therapy and, as time went by, it became a course which I taught to therapists who wanted to deal with weight issue clients.

The trouble was that all the people I really wanted to reach were not going to fit into my clinic; and all the information you needed to have, was not going to fit into a one week course.

So, with support and unconditional love from my Mother, the inherited sense of justice, obsession and workaholic nature from my most wonderful, now departed Father, this book came to life.

Other corners of my life had to do a pincer movement to get me to a place where I could write this. There was the irritation and faith from the Greek element in my life, Spyros, and also a very dear old friend, Duncan Turner, who has stuck with me through all the trials and tantrums!

My thanks go to all the friends, clients and associates who pushed me to write this and, of course, Bruce Farrow, mentor and friend and the very inimitable Steve Richards, my publisher, who prodded me into action!

So, my thanks, love and affection to you.

Be well, be free and, most of all,

Be you.

Chapter 1

They don't want you to have it! Why?

Welcome to the diet book which everyone in the diet industry will probably hate! Why? Well, the whole reason for writing this is to give you the tools to get the look you want and to be able to use the diet, ethos and other bits of information on an ongoing basis PLUS cheat and be a rebel once a week. This is the unique and effective way to keep your metabolism raised plus give you the freedom to live your life.

The 'rebelling' basically means that you don't have to diet seven days a week – you can incorporate the diet into your lifestyle as and when you need to. You also have your *Rebel Diet* day, which is a major cheat day and also has a few other stipulations with it, like have fun, do something for you, do something you have never done before, but of most all...REBEL! Rebel against the diet industry, Rebel against the constraints of life and Rebel against what you 'should' be doing!

What is simple about dieting?
It's not a mystery, not the Holy Grail, and not some secret to which only a few people hold the key – regardless of what the gurus charging vast amounts per hour tell you. Dieting IS straight forward once you understand the principles and get to know your own body.

What is not simple is dealing with the rest of life, mental motivation, self-confidence and image problems which help or hinder your efforts in being the person you want to be. If you don't feel like changing and don't have the motivation to do it for *you* then there's not a single diet or pill that will work.

Welcome to the world of dealing with the whole person, as well as an effective and revolutionary new diet system and attitude. Welcome to *Rebel Diet*.

You may want to just skip to the diet pages, which is fine, although you will find that others who read the book throughout have better long-term results as they will gain all the tips, knowledge and understanding to get the most out of the system and ethos.

So, why does this work?

Well, there are a number of reasons why, if we want to lose weight, we can't just do it.

Obviously there are medical reasons for some, but others can't find the drive to do it because nothing works for them; they diet for a while and then fall off the wagon, or find it so restrictive that they can't have a 'life' and generally resent the world and all within it.

Also, if you don't believe you are worth it, not good enough or will never succeed at anything, then nothing will work for you either. Oh, maybe for the short term or in bursts, but then this just creates a serial dieter which is not helpful for the mind, confidence or body.

Again, this is where this book is very different. From working with clients over many years, it has been evident to me that if someone doesn't have the drive to do it for 'themselves' then anything they wish to achieve will never happen.

Within the book are chapters about self-esteem, body image and confidence which are aimed to help you increase your own self-confidence and personal strength throughout the diet and really begin to enjoy the benefits of what you are doing, not only in seeing results in your body, but also your mental attitude which flows into other areas of your life.

Have you noticed that, when you feel low, nothing really feels worth it? Sometimes you lose interest in how you look and everything seems like it's either 'too much' or 'too difficult'?

It's time to reclaim 'you', the person you always knew you could be. Not just externally, but internally too. While building the internal 'you' up, the external 'you' and image begins to change with a very simple diet routine and some very simple exercise guidelines; these guidelines change as you change and adapt as your body reacts to each stage of dieting.

This isn't some tree-hugging, madcap idea – it's based on how the signalling from the brain affects our physical reactions, the rate our metabolism works at and how the structure of our mental and emotional state can change our body's efficiency. It might sound a bit technical, it's all explained in simple terms through the book.

So, let's rebel against those restrictive diets, rebel against the diet industry, rebel against constraints holding you back and rebel against dieting seven days a week!

The diet itself is designed so that you have a structured start to it. That way, you get to know your body and how it responds to various parts of the diet, like high and low carbohydrate days. When you recognise those telltale signs you begin to know exactly how to kick-start your body into responding again when things slow down; eventually you will just implement the diet when you need to and know exactly what to do.

Easy...well, yes.

No more expensive meals from special diet companies, no more endless searches for 'the answer'. This isn't rocket science.

How do you think I managed to get to know exactly what to do with my own diet to keep body fat off? How do you think so many other athletes and people 'in the know' manage their weight when potentially they have a weight problem? We simply got to know our system and what to do when.

Contained in the book are useful tips on rapid weight loss. This is when you need to drop a couple of pounds overnight and fit into that dress. It's not actually body fat loss but excess water loss; it's one of those secrets that the diet industry tends to use in the early stages of a diet to make you believe you have lost weight when in fact you are no longer retaining excess water.

Now, the concept of having a cheat day may terrify you, but I can assure you from my own experience of competing and dieting that the day after your cheat day, your Rebel Day, is when your body fat loss is kicked up a notch.

An Overall Rebel

Most people have no idea which way to turn for practical help which they can incorporate into their lifestyle.

One thing that becomes really clear as you diet and try to get that stubborn weight to move is that you are in fact unique and will therefore respond differently to everyone else. That's why standard diets don't work long-term – they aren't tailored to YOU!

If you happen to have a stubborn system then you may well have a slow metabolism.

This could be due to a number of internal factors which just relate to your own body make-up, or could also be due to a number of external factors to do with your lifestyle, stress, time, no loo roll and many other things which will affect you.

The *Rebel Diet* is constructed so that you can:

1) Identify the problems which affect your body fat loss; and
2) Be able to change them when you need or want to. It's all about YOU.

We aren't saints, we will sometimes have our off days, we will sometimes fall off the wagon – so why not use that time the way it SHOULD be used? We don't want you to FALL off the wagon – we're going to PUSH you off!

Why?
Well, for many reasons which will become apparent throughout this manual, but the MAIN one is to get your metabolism running faster, as well as:

1) Having fun whilst reducing stress, which is a major factor in weight loss;
2) Getting a break from the prison of a regular diet regime;
3) Building on 'you' and your ability to succeed (building self-confidence); and
4) Providing constant momentum to change your whole life around in the long term.

So, forget about the lack of motivation from long term dieting. Forget about the strict regimes, and let's get some time back for you and grab that drive and confidence you know you have! Sort out some of those problems that hinder the success you know you can have.

This is a simple manual which will teach you how to speed up your metabolism and make changes which will help you achieve the look you want and to keep it going.

There is no right or wrong – if you want to come off the diet for a bit, then that's fine. If you decide you need to put it back in place, then that's fine too. It all comes down to your own perspective and beliefs about your own capabilities.

Beliefs are like self-fulfilling prophecies, so whether you believe you can or you cannot – you are absolutely right. Let's believe that you *can*. Let's give you the tools to take charge and root out those difficulties which are not giving you what you want.

The *Rebel Diet's* entire system is dedicated to explaining why those problems occur, to let you see them coming and solve them, thus ensuring a three-pronged approach to change.

They all look like stick insects!
You aren't on your own. The most unlikely people you know or see every day may have or have had problems which relate to eating or weight. Don't be fooled by seeing people who are not overweight and assume they have everything under control. So many people work very hard at keeping the weight off so never think you are the only one, even though at times it may feel like it. It's just that they've found what works for *them* and so will you.

Rebel Diet: Freeing You from Diet Hell

The Smiling Shit Philosophy

Society, career, social expectations and image all create this prison of behaviour that is expected of us and if you don't fit into that mould you are an outsider. Recognise that?

Let's make this work for *you*, be proud of who you are and the fact that you don't fit in that box. My Father once told me that sometimes outwardly-rebelling meets with defensive opposition so, in those cases, you have to become a 'smiling shit'. He said that even though you are still rebelling and intending on changing something fundamental, there is less opposition and hard work if you change it from within and become a 'stealth smiling shit'!.

Our society and lifestyle has changed dramatically over the years and the pressure on us to conform and to be a success is immense. Gone are the days of being 'happy with our lot', while the praise and social fondness of the 'eccentric' have been replaced with a belittling of the ethos of being an individual.

Time, stress, family, and social and career pressures have changed the way we live and even the most straightforward of lifestyles can be pressurised. All this has a knock-on effect on the way we feel about ourselves and can lead us to question whether we are really good enough if we don't reach the perceived standards which have been set by the media.

If you change your shape or size because you feel you *should* so that you can fit in, then I ask you to read through the mental change chapter of this book. Also, if you feel you 'should' then it is unlikely you will ever succeed, as it isn't for you. If you feel you *want* to – then you will.

Some of my clients have found that when we do the groundwork of changes to their own self-confidence, self-belief and success, they in fact decide that they *are* happy with how they look and bollocks to everyone else who thinks they should change. All of a sudden I see a person blossom and revel in their own individuality and feel comfortable about how they look. At this point I usually tell them about the 'smiling shit' before they go out and start locking antlers with everyone, and suddenly they start to see the changes they can make in various situations like their career, family, personal relationships, projects etc, quietly and with the path of least resistance, and are completely amazed.

If, on the other hand, you know you *want* to change your shape or size then that is totally different. If you know that, when you *do* make the change, you will feel better and more 'you' then you have come to the right place and I look forward to the various sensations and revelations you will experience on your journey.

Remember – we all need to rebel in some way, so let's make it fun and make it work for you.

Rebel Nuts and Bolts
The *Rebel Diet Revolution* is a demystified diet, broken down into sections for you to use at the times you need to.

To make this work really well, this manual takes you through the steps of getting to know your own body and what speeds up and slows down your system.

You can use the diets in the manual when you need to and when you recognise that you should; you can also exercise if you want to (there is a guide for exercise here too). But, most importantly, you can make changes in your body shape and also in your life at the same time.

The background information before getting to the nitty gritty diet section is all about other things that affect your ability to lose weight and is aimed to help keep up the motivation, which is hugely important.

This isn't just about weight loss; it's also about increasing your own self esteem, confidence and quality of life which, in fact, all go hand in hand.

Increasing self-esteem and confidence from being able to follow and implement this diet system into your busy life will give you a feeling of achievement. This then helps further confidence as you see yourself change, believe in yourself and your ability to do those things that you want to do in your life. On top of that, your improved self-image gives you that extra boost to get out there and do all the things you wanted to do. Oh, then of course you have increased energy from the additional confidence and weight loss and so it keeps on going.

Most of us have experienced times or know someone who has tried really hard to lose weight. They buy a book or see a diet, buy all the right foods, take out a gym membership, get started…but then lose motivation, cheat and then quit totally. Once they stop they put the weight back on, plus a bit more, and feel absolutely terrible because they feel they have failed!

I Don't Want You To Be Like Me
This diet has been developed to work for EVERYONE.

One of the points raised is that people, mostly women, are worried that they will end up looking like me from a muscular point of view. However, most people want to know how I keep the body fat low. What they don't realise is that I have a predisposition to putting on fat because of my naturally sluggish metabolic rate.

The assumption is that because I keep the body fat low, I don't have a problem. If I was to laugh every time I heard that, I would probably offend lots of people, even though I do have an immense talent for offending some people, especially if they are officious prats!

Rebel Diet: Freeing You from Diet Hell

Let's knock a few myths on the head here and now! My physique is as a result of the following:

- Over twenty years of hard training
- Years of competing at international level
- Five days a week of strictly maintained training devised from getting to know my body and understanding what I respond to and what I don't
- Drive and passion for my sport
- Learning from many mistakes along the way and constantly working on technique to produce the best World Record-producing results.

So, you will not look like me – that is, you will not put on muscle from a diet. My physique is from training and competing for over twenty years and the last thing most of you want to do is have any muscle – that's why nowhere in this book is there anything on weight training, just toning.

This is a manual for body fat loss – if you want to tone, then I will shortly be offering a totally different book purely for toning, firming and tightening up.

Remember, my physique is not created just from wishing to look like this. It is a by-product of competing at a high standard for years which creates a muscular physique. The amount of times I have been invited to appear on TV shows to discuss why I *want* to look like this is deeply irritating.

I remember an agent I had for a while who rang me, all excited, as someone from GMTV wanted me on to do a piece on why 'I push myself to create my physique'. Now, even after I explained to both the agent and the GMTV representative that I never intended to be as muscular, I just happened to look like this from competing for so long and the amount of heavy training I had put in over the years, I still got another phone call from the agent asking me to reconsider. I vividly remember the mouthful of coffee I was having at the time spraying the terracotta wall in front of me!

It goes without saying that she didn't stay my agent for very long.

Working on *The Trisha Show* was different. The wonderful thing about having worked with *The Trisha Show* was that they understood first and foremost that I was a specialist therapist and that I also trained therapists. They also understood and appreciated my long-term research and experience of dealing with weight and eating related issues and never batted an eyelid about my physique; they knew that my own competing was something separate to the work I did.

On the one hand it was wonderful as I could just get on with my job, yet on the other hand I did wonder if I was losing my presence! I was lucky to have been given people to work with who were really desperate for change and the results they experienced were wonderful, which is certainly gratifying for me to see.

So, I also hope you are now armed with the correct information to deal with any ignorant comments you hear about other female athletes, e.g. Dame Kelly Homes, Fatima Whitbread and many more hard-working athletes.

Shall I get off my soapbox now?!

So, here we go. Let's take the first steps in changing the way you look, your self-esteem and hopefully elements of your goals - and all for the better.

Remember, weight management isn't just about diet - it's about You and Your Life. You are unique and being unique makes you special with a right to your own individuality, beliefs and values.

This is for you.

'I do not wish to be a common man!
Be it my right to be uncommon.
I can seek opportunity – not security!
I want to take calculated risks, to dream and to build,
to fail and succeed.
I will never cower before any master, nor bend to any threat!'

Franklin D Roosevelt

Chapter 2

The Diet Industry

The diet industry is a multi-million pound industry.

How much money do you think you have spent on diets, pills, specific diet meals and courses and possibly books? Hundreds, maybe even thousands?

Have any of them worked for you long term?

The diet industry has made fortunes out of turning the very simple basics of weight loss into a complete mystery by selling various pills and compounds, or by selling expensive processed meals which you can prepare yourself at a fraction of the price.

There seems to have been a mysterious veil drawn up around dieting when in fact it is very simple indeed. The only difficult part of changing your body shape and body fat levels is knowing what works for you and how to find out. Also, many diets are not sustainable long term as they can cause repeated severe dieting and you can end up gaining more weight than you started off with!

The Secret?
There isn't a secret. It's all about understanding your own system and how to tweak it to make you lose weight.

In the past, we didn't have the convenience we have now and generally people were a lot more active. Shops were not as close, more people had to walk and entertainment involved having to go out.

We pretty much had to make our own entertainment and there were fewer home-based activities. Having a car was not as common as it is now. Everyone now has a car and those people who can't drive are few and far between.

Our food was better; there was less processed food and more cooked from scratch with natural produce. A lot of the food was locally produced (especially where I was brought up in Belfast where, at that time, a Kiwi fruit was thought of as highly exotic!). Pre-cooked and processed convenience food was more of a luxury than an every day occurrence.

Many companies sprang up and began to offer potions, pills and diet solutions, some of them were effective, some of them not so effective, but very few of them actually offered a long-term solution to managing your weight. It was about short term weight loss and was not designed for your own body. Where would the profit be in giving people a long term solution that did not generate repeat business?

The way the industry seems to be working at the moment is this:

- They give you absolutely no information and they hold the key to the 'secret'; or
- They give you apparently lots of information, just not quite enough to be able to do it yourself - but will sell you all the meals; or
- They give you all the information based on 'normal' people, and don't give the variants needed for those who don't fit into the 'normal' category.

Many of the diets which are around are based on short term, fast solutions which don't keep the weight off long term. It's all part of the quick fix, 'want it now' society we seem to have grown into. It doesn't have to be like that – it's simple and easy. And do you know what? The less you stress about it the better the long term results.

Even apart from what I have written, you will probably know certain things that do work for you or you respond well to.

One piece of advice I can give you is that when you find something you respond well to, you can incorporate it into the regime in the book in some way AND USE IT! It will be an indicator of what you respond to and then you are on your way to recognising the signals which get you closer to understanding what your body needs and when.

I'm not going to say that my way is the only way, as we are all individual, but the key is getting to know your body and metabolism and to bring all the elements together.

Diet Pills

This is a tricky subject. I will have to be careful what I say here unless I want a ream of paperwork from lawyers all threatening lawsuits!

As far as I am concerned, there is a place for everything. They can be useful when your metabolic rate has really slowed and can assist is pushing you through a plateau. However, there are much easier and less costly ways of doing this.

Amphetamine and natural derivatives

Many of the diet pills available are based on speeding up your metabolism which will cause some stress on the body. There are a number of downfalls with this, as you are essentially artificially speeding up your system with a thermogenic effect. This means that you will feel warmer as your metabolism increases.

The problem with using pills instead of naturally speeding metabolism up through timings of meals, is that when you stop taking them your metabolic rate then drops back and you get a slow down and weight tends to go back on UNLESS YOU STAY ON THEM.

If you do stay on them, then your body gets used to it and you need to up the dosage. They will generally help you with alertness, a feeling of more energy and therefore add to weight loss; however, long term usage can cause problems and in fact increase weight in the long run.

They can have a long term detrimental side effect, especially if they are essentially amphetamine or pseudo amphetamine-based. Examples of these are:

1) *Guarana*

Commonly marketed. If you do buy it you need to make sure it is from a pure source, as so many places now manufacture it and mix in ingredients to fill it out. Guarana is from Brazil. It comes from a pretty fruit-bearing plant and the bit that is used is the seed inside the fruit. The seed is ground down and then used as a natural stimulant in tablet, drink and a kind of strange food form! The reason why it works is that the caffeine content is three times the strength of coffee beans.

2) *Caffeine Tablets & T5*

Well now, we all know about these. Caffeine tablets have been around in one form or another for some time. As with all stimulants, they can work for a while then you need to increase the dosage and eventually burn the system out over time. You can gain the same increase in energy and metabolic rate over a period if you change your diet and timings, etc - it just takes a bit longer and is much safer longer term without the side effects.

Note: T5 (also known as ECA) is a combination of caffeine, ephedrine or ephedra and aspirin. The caffeine is for speeding up your system, the ephedrine is for the same thing and the aspirin is used for getting it into your system much more quickly and effectively. Not a good combination, with side effects of elevated blood pressure, palpitations, sweating, nausea and can also lead to anxiety in some cases.[1]

---

[1] Adverse Effects of Botanical and Non-Botanical Ephedrine Products by June Weintraub, Harvard University, USA.

Ephedra
Ephedra refers to the name of the plant it is harvested from. It is also know as Ma Huang. It has a pseudoephedrine and ephedrine content and so is a stimulant and also a thermogenic. It has been used in decongestants and in respiratory illnesses for many years. Again, the side effects can include elevated blood pressure, anxiety, palpitations, sweating, nausea and seizures.[2] Long term usage is really not advised, so isn't it better to have a system in place which will give you the results you want without all of the complications?

At the time of writing, ephedra was illegal to sell over the counter but the inclusion of ephedra in restricted doses of dietary supplements was allowable. However, this changes on a regular basis. Let's just say there are better ways of getting your system to speed up without needing to use stimulants.

Growth Hormone, GH, HGH
Ah, now here is something which is all the rage. Commonly called 'the elixir of youth'. Yes, it is true that using growth hormones can have an added side effect of burning body fat due to the change of utilisation of glycogen in the body. However, for it to work properly for body fat loss, it requires a number of other systems to be in place along with a number of other chemicals which include certain types of steroids. Even if you were tempted by the adverts out there about GH, here are a few facts:

1) Growth Hormone is a living organism.
2) It has to still be 'alive' in the terms of a working liquid compound when administered.
3) It can only be kept 'alive' by keeping it at a certain temperature and not disrupted by vigorous movement.
4) For maximum effect it needs to be administered subcutaneously (there is an argument whether it is subcutaneously or intramuscular) which involves it being injected.
5) It cannot be ingested and then transported through the system internally.
6) It comes in measurements of 'IU'.
7) Real Growth Hormone can only be prescribed. It is sold on the black market and the costs are between £150 and £300 per 60IU. It is VERY expensive and the black market is so flooded with fake GH that many people have stopped trying to buy it unless they can

---
[2] Memorial Sloan-Kettering Cancer Centre research 2007.

find a dodgy doctor to prescribe it for them if they do not medically need it.

The point I am making is that many places are selling what they claim to be Growth Hormone in a tablet, nasal spray or gel form and jumping on the band wagon with it, just because it has been reported on the news as being a 'wonder drug'. All they need is one in 50 of us to buy one of the products once at £30 or £40 per product, when we then realise it doesn't work after trying it, and they have a very healthy short term profit. So, when you see products claiming to be Growth Hormone, bear in mind what GH really is, what form it has to be in to be able to work, as well as the costs of the real stuff. You will be able to work out pretty quickly what is bogus and designed to get a quick buck out of you.

Appetite suppressants are another one. There are various ways that these work, but what happens when you stop? Again, the system has been hyped up, the body has been put under stress, and it all slows down when you stop taking them. Then what happens when you start eating properly again and your metabolism slows down? Is it worth it?

There are lots of other products on the market that all claim to do amazing things, and some do have their place along with a good diet and exercise regime.

However, why pay for something chemical which you will have to stay on indefinitely? Quite frankly, if there was something which really worked, was safe and had no long term side effects then we would all be using it. We would have no weight problems and there would be no point in writing this book!

There are some natural herbal supplements which can aid the platform of effective body function and therefore better utilisation of body fat, and I have included them at the end of this book. However, be aware that none of them are a 'miracle' and, as they are herbal, quite frequently have a number of research papers about them either saying they work or they don't. They can work if used in combination with an effective diet and a bit of exercise, but they will not be the answer to your prayers simply used on their own.

Short Term Rapid Weight Loss Diets
These include the cabbage soup diet, melon diet, and all forms of dramatic weight loss, short term diets.

Well, first of all, the initial rapid weight loss you have is from the reduction of carbohydrate. When this happens the body sheds the excess water which gives you the sudden drop in weight initially. You think 'wow, this really works'!

So, from basically being starved you will lose some weight and body fat. The problem is, your poor old system thinks you are starving it to death, goes into panic mode and slows down your metabolic rate to conserve energy and generally becomes very efficient.

Once you have come off the short term diet, even though you lost weight, when you start increasing the carbohydrates again, you will get some water retention and that horrible, bloated feeling. Then, as if that wasn't bad enough, because the body has slowed the metabolism, you don't burn off what you eat as quickly so you have a predisposition to putting on weight again. A lot of people end up putting more weight back on than they lost.

You may have dropped two dress sizes very quickly but, when you are done, the weight may have gone back and possibly a bit more. You feel rubbish, you don't like how you look and the only person apparently to blame is you.

Not so! If you had just enough information on what to do once you had dropped the weight and understood why certain stages were working, then you could have continued and maintained the weight loss. So, it wasn't you that was at fault at all. It's the provider's responsibility to aftercare.

Low or No Carbohydrate Diets
As the name suggests, low or no carbohydrate diets demand a severe reduction of carbohydrates. But this will in fact have a detrimental effect on your system and you may well find it increasingly harder to keep body fat levels down. Great results short term, but over time it is very difficult to maintain.

Really strict dieting over a long period of time and restriction of fats and other essential nutrients not only weakens your immune system and slows your metabolism, but it also makes you more likely to cheat: it reduces your motivation as you see the body fat loss slow down. It creates doubt about your ability to stick to a diet and to get the look you want for yourself. This also has a big impact on your self-esteem and self-confidence. That is NOT what this is about.

If your belief in yourself and your own ability to lose weight and to stick to a diet is in question, then anything which seems like it isn't working will further impact on your motivation to carry on and so you lose confidence and motivation.

If, for instance, you understood what your body was doing when your fat loss slowed down, would that de-motivate you or would you then know what to do and be able to get it moving again?

Simply by understanding what is happening with your body and what other outside situations affect it, you can change your diet regime and lose or maintain quite easily. This in turn starts a chain reaction, gaining confidence from seeing something you want actually happen. Then the feel good factor of being able to see the changes in you starts to trickle into other areas of your life and soon you notice how much more confident you are in new and current projects and goals. It really does make a difference to your entire wellbeing.

At the time of writing I am coming up to competition and in fact dieting right now to lose half a stone to make my weight category. As always, the more I stress about it the less I lose so, right now, I am thinking 'to hell with it, I'll just weigh in over my limit'. As a result, my weight is coming down!

Look – I want you to take this information, use it and learn how to incorporate it into your life to use when and if you need it. Simple.

At the same time, if you can improve your self-esteem, rebel against the system and show everyone you can do anything you decide to do, then that is even better!!!

You just need the formulas of what to do and when.

'Behind every successful man is a surprised woman'
Maryon Pearson

Chapter 3

Understanding You & The Stress Monsters

You are completely unique
No one else has your life. No one knows your thoughts, knows how you react to things, or knows how you really see yourself.

Your body is also completely unique – it responds to your emotions, the stresses around it, what you put in it and how you look after it. It works at its own natural speed, repairs itself and operates in a way which is totally individual to you.

So, if we are all so individual, why would we have Body Mass Index and Basal Metabolic Rate calculators which are available everywhere?

Apparently these are all based on a 'normal' person

Now, defining what is actually 'normal' is a bit of a difficult question. Normal according to whom?

Does this normal person weigh 8 stone, never put on any body fat and is 5ft 3in tall? Or are they 6ft 7in and weigh 26 stone?

I would love to meet this 'normal' person. That normal person would need to have the same bone density, the same metabolism, muscle mass, body fat distribution and water levels as all the rest of us for them to be useful in any way in creating an index to decide if we are overweight or not.

For instance, a person who naturally carry a dense physique, more muscle and heavier bone structure will naturally weigh heavier than someone else who has exactly the same dimensions but will probably be shown as overweight on the body mass index (BMI), whereas the other person may be shown to be within 'acceptable levels'.

Let me give you an example – ME!

Now, as you know I compete. I try to keep my body fat levels reasonably low and, for a woman, I am very muscular.

So – muscle is heavier than body fat (due to the density). My weight is around 86kgs or 190lbs. According to the BMI, I am obese for my height of 5ft 7in. Does that make any sense? Answers on a postcard…

One thing I have learnt over the years is that <u>everything depends on:</u>

1) How your system operates – metabolism, response to different levels of exercise, foods etc.
2) The current situation in your life – stress, depression, pressure form work and family etc., and how your body reacts to it.

This is all unique to you

I can remember getting ready for bodybuilding competitions and having various so-called 'gurus' working with me. They couldn't understand why I had stopped losing body fat when all the other people they had worked with would have already got down to 5% body fat and be ready for competition.

These 'gurus' never asked me about what had happened before when I dieted. In fact, they never even asked me how long I had been dieting or any of the other questions which give you a warning that your metabolic rate has slowed.

So, over a period of time I started working with my own system and began to help others who were having the same problems as me.

A client that I worked with phoned me once to say that she had put on a kilo in weight but had gone *down* a dress size and was panicking. She had been on diets for so long that, when she started doing the *Rebel Diet*, her body soaked up all the nutrients that were going in, her metabolism sped up and burnt more body fat. However, because the body tissue was more dense as a result of actually having what it needed, she weighed slightly heavier.

Remember – we all have different goals, lifestyles and stress levels, but there are still the same old things which affect our bodies and cause us weight problems.

I still work with athletes as well as people who don't train, who have trouble getting down to their target weight. Every person comes along with his or her own unique set of circumstances.

Realistically, they don't really need me now, but I suppose sometimes you just want someone to tell you what to do!

In fact, for my own diet, I write it down on a piece of paper and give it to someone else to give back to me! It's as though someone else has written it for me and that way I know I will put everything into it!

Strange but true, but I thought you might like to know that this author has had most of the problems she is writing about!

This is one of the things I am here for
Suddenly realising that no one else had the answer apart from me was a turning point. Taking the responsibility for change onto myself and not looking for anyone else to give me the answers was like a freedom and is

now one of the keys of success I have had with so many clients.

Getting to know and understanding your own body and becoming aware of why it is reacting in certain ways and adapting to it is your absolute key.

I'm just helping you with a few short cuts so it doesn't take as long for you to get the formula!

The mental side of dieting

This is a hugely important factor which never gets discussed. In fact, it is totally ignored even though it is a crucial part of your success or failure with your bodyweight.

Let's put it this way. Stress, as you know, can cause you to lose a lot of weight very quickly. A traumatic shock can send the body into mayhem and trigger the 'survival' system which is to increase adrenaline and operate on the level you need to survive and get through what has happened. It is also part of the fight or flight reaction.

However, if it persists and you are still operating on a 'stressed' level, then it becomes chronic and can lead to adrenal burnout and also a drop in metabolic rate for protection. Addressing the issues in your life can vastly improve the physical response you get when you want to diet, compete, climb Mount Everest or whatever.

Your emotional state, as you know, creates various chemical reactions in the brain which then filter through to the body and, depending on what that emotional state is, will produce varying physiological effects.

So, in short, your mental and emotional state will have a direct effect on your results in dieting or any other goals you wish to achieve. If you don't believe you can do it, if you don't have belief in yourself, have self-confidence or esteem issues, then it will all have a knock-on effect on your ability to achieve, particularly in relation to things you want to achieve for YOU.

Your emotional state from other factors in your life can also directly affect your physical performance. Have you noticed how, when you are feeling good, you can achieve so much, simply because you believe in what you are doing and you physically feel ready to take on the challenge?

Conversely, when you feel down, you don't feel capable of anything and are possibly physically tired and run down?

Nothing can happen if you don't have a head. What I mean is, all physical responses have to come from the brain. It is the brain which gives the signals and commands for everything in your body to happen, so, when you don't happen to have a head, you tend to die! Right?

In other words, if your situation and mental wellbeing is at its optimal level, then your body will operate at an optimal level too. If there are other reactions going on, like reacting to stress, depression etc., then the straight signals become convoluted with all the other protection mechanisms kicking in and being initiated form the brain to the body, so the signals then become less effective when you are trying to achieve something.

For all the changes you want to make, for everything you want to succeed in, look at how you feel right now. If you are not in the best emotional place right now then this is the time to start making the changes. It doesn't have to be major and it will clear the path to success.

Some emotional states also have a direct effect on us physically, which restricts our results in weight issues and body fat loss. So, the last thing I want to do is to create a diet system which will stress you out, make you feel imprisoned, restricted, depress you, cause you trauma or result in anything which will hamper your results.

Not only would it be unfair on you, it would also not do me any good!

This is one of the areas where the *Rebel Diet* is different. It addresses what mental states affect the body and helps you to not only successfully change your shape but, also gives you the resources to change your mental and emotional wellbeing. This, in turn, will produce an optimum physical reaction and, hopefully, also create a more compelling future for you.

So, let's have a look at a few negative mental states which affect dieting:

Stress and Dieting
Ah, our old friend stress!! I suppose I do harp on about stress, but that's because it is the most common element which puts a spanner in the works.

By stress, I do not really mean the stress that happens immediately after a major trauma. However, to explain what happens at this point is useful in giving an insight into your long term stress problem.

When we have a trauma, there is frequently a major stress element for a short period afterwards (I am not referring to chronic long term stress here, that's coming up!).

At that moment, we go into a safety procedure to protect ourselves and the body responds by producing that wonderful stuff called adrenaline into our bodies.

At this point we operate on almost an automatic pilot mode and the fight or flight mechanism kicks in. You may also have noticed at this point, that there isn't a lot of emotion until AFTER the event has happened.

Our metabolic rate is increased, we are sharp, reactive, focused and our body is in a high state of alert in survival mode.

If you have stress over a long a period of time after an event, or are continuing in a stressful situation over a long period of time, this then becomes very tiring mentally and physically.

Mentally you are still operating in that raised awareness and it is very difficult to focus on anything else, decision-making on other subjects can be confused or you feel that you are procrastinating or wandering around in a great big fog.

Sometimes, during these periods, the ability to think clearly about other issues outside of the stressful situation seems to be impaired. So, personal decisions about your future, relationships or even simple daily tasks can be difficult to cope with and trying to move your life forward can seem daunting.

The physical response to the mental state is to slow the metabolism down eventually after the initial shock, as this preserves the body. Also, the adrenaline, which is possibly still being produced at a higher level, can produce adrenal burnout and lower the metabolism even more. A feeling of fatigue, lethargy, lowered self esteem and lack of motivation can occur.

Long term stress has also shown to be a contributing factor to heart problems and immune system deficiencies as well as various other physiological symptoms like skin irritations, hair loss, ulcers and digestive system disorders.

Stress doesn't have to be from one major event. It can be a lifestyle issue as well. Demands on our time expectations, work and personal issues can all build on each other to culminate in what feels like a great weight sitting on your head. It's like building blocks, one stacking on the other until the point when even the tiniest of blocks can send the entire construction tumbling to the ground.

When you have been under stress, did you notice that when you addressed and dealt with just one or two elements of that stress and resolved them, how much better you felt? How much more positive you felt? How much did your outlook and motivation change in order to deal with other areas of your life?

Even if you are stuck in a situation which is unlikely to change and you are in a position where you can't do anything about it, you can still change how you react to it.

The only person who can make the decision about how you react to and feel about any situation is YOU.

No one else can teach you or force you to feel that way. That decision has to come from you at a very basic level. Even though it may feel like we are forced into feeling a particular way about something, or someone 'made me feel bad', in reality, that decision was made by you.

For instance, when you drive a car, the only person who can decide where you are going is you. You may have been instructed to go a certain way or to have to be somewhere at a particular time, but the only person who makes the decisions at that time and turns the wheel, puts their foot on the accelerator or brake, is YOU. The only person actually driving that car is you.

A lot of how we feel about things is a conditioned response to react in a certain way, which again is completely controlled by you. No one else is inside your head making that decision for you. It is your decision.

Dissociative Technique
If you are deciding to change how you feel about a situation which is immovable, then just take a step outside the situation. See it as though you were watching a movie and see yourself in the movie.

Notice what the others are doing, how they feel, why they react the way they do from their childhood, life experiences, values and beliefs and you will see the situation in a different perspective. As you do that, ask yourself, 'What is it that I need to learn from this situation or event, the learning of which will allow me to let go of the stress and negative emotion? What can I see when I look at this as it really is, not how I perceive and feel it to be?'

This is part of a highly effective major technique which I use with clients. It is only a very small part but highly effective. The reason that it works is that when we are 'in' a situation, often it is very hard to be objective about it; it's almost like being sucked into an emotional vortex.

The technique allows you to step outside the situation, to look at it clinically which will resolve negative emotions, stress etc., associated with that event or situation.

Once you do that, often options become clear; you understand a part of something which previously was stressing you out and puts it into a completely new perspective. This assists you in being able to dissociate from the problem and frees you up to make new choices, giving positive movement towards WHAT YOU WANT.

If you are under stress of any kind, then motivation, focus, confidence and clarity of thought may be an issue and would certainly affect you ability to keep to a diet or even make you feel that it's not worth doing for yourself. You may also feel that it's too much to take on.

That is why:

1) You can deal with small elements of stress and build on the confidence that you CAN resolve things and gain more confidence from it.
2) Benefit from the feeling of achievement in dealing with a stress

element as well as losing weight. It builds momentum, rolling into other areas of your life. It's very infectious!
3) You can tackle one of the stress elements, and start small. Just pick one small thing and deal with it. Notice how good you feel and then choose the next thing.
4) The *Rebel Diet* is designed to give you freedom. You can implement it when you want to or need to, so there is never a 'feeling of failure' element to it. In fact, you are FORCED to cheat once a week!
5) You need to deal with stress which affects you physically and mentally and hinders your progress and results from dieting.

Dieting and Depression
Depression is something which happens in varying degrees.

Many of us describe ourselves as being 'depressed' when in fact we are just bit under the weather.

A real proper humdinger of a depression has severe implications on our daily ability for dealing with simple life tasks; it can affect our relationships with others and, of course, severely affect our self belief, confidence and motivation.

We all have our off days and one of the things we frequently don't do is allow ourselves to have an 'off' day. Again, the pressure on us to be perfect and wonderful all the time is actually pretty high. I'm not quite sure when all of a sudden we were supposed to be fabulous all the time and people's general ability to let us have a 'bad hair day' went out the window.

Believe it or not, many people put themselves under pressure to always be tolerant and 'perfect'; however, this can build up huge amounts of anger and resentment which colour our view of how we see the world and everyone in it dramatically.

This, then, also affects our objectivity on many situations or relationships we have, not only with others, but also with ourselves.

Low self esteem and light to moderate depression also contribute to seeing ourselves in a bad light. The image we have in our head and what we see in the mirror can be greatly distorted, and the belief that we can succeed in what we set our minds to can also suffer.

When you are having a low day or a low period, there are options on how to deal with it. You can either decide to save it to the Rebel Day and wallow in it for that day, along with raiding the local pastry shop; OR you can look at your watch, decide to take maybe 10 minutes or even an hour, and have a really good bad hair day for that period of time. Set yourself a limit to the time you will dedicate to that.

The reasons why this works are:

1) You are allowed to have the time to feel low.
2) You are allowed to have moments when you don't feel great as you are in fact human.
3) It dedicates an allotted time to feeling that way instead of feeling like you have to fight it off, in which case it stagnates and drags on over a longer period.
4) It makes that time specific to you and your needs.

This is all for light depression times or low moments. For more serious depression, here is a different scenario.

I had a client who was very overweight, approximately 26 stone, 5ft 7in tall and seriously clinically depressed. He slept most of the day, would not go out, was so low in self-confidence that he was ashamed to be seen in public because of what he thought others would think of him. He had lost a great deal of self-belief because of the situation he had ended up in.

There were a number of things he could not do. He found it hard to bathe or shower; due to his inactivity, his mobility was greatly reduced; he pushed friends and family away because of how he felt about himself.

So the first thing to do was to give him small things to do for himself. Now, the key with severe depression is to understand that what seems like very insignificant steps to us, are major milestones to others, so accomplishing very little things begins to gently build self-confidence and motivation.

We started with the famous 'Dynobands'. They have been around for many years and have been the saviour of many in rehabilitation and so many other situations. Unfortunately, the Stage 1 Dynoband is in fact pink which doesn't please many male clients!

So, simply by doing some light exercises each morning and evening for 20 minutes and slightly changing his diet, including the infamous Rebel Day, he began to see what he could achieve. He also noticed quickly a change in his physique and the weight initially rapidly began to come off.

As this was happening, his own self-perception improved and he began to go out more, see his friends and family more, and didn't worry so much about how he thought others saw him.

Of course, that initial great weight loss slowed down but, because he understood what was happening, he dealt with it with help from the diet section which is in the book, and kept it going. That was another success for him. He was doing it on his own and taking control of his life.

It was all a chain reaction and gradually, over time, he lost weight. He got back to work and has changed his entire life around. I am so very proud of him that I don't have the words to describe it.

So, simply by taking very small steps, and I mean *really* small steps, and making no apology for it to others, he turned severe clinical depression around over the period of a year and turned his life around with it at the same time. Now, many people are on anti-depressant medication in these sorts of situations which, if prescribed correctly, can help enormously.

One thing which has always been hammered home to me by people in the medical profession and researchers is that if you are not happy with any medication or are worried about how you feel on it, then always go back to your doctor and ask. Even if it 'just doesn't feel right', just check with your doctor. If you don't tell them then how can they ever know and be able to fix it for you?

Don't start taking it into your own hands – talk to your doctor. If you get to the stage where you want to come off anti-depressants, then a simple discussion will help you plan on how to come off them and what to expect.

Some anti-depressants can speed up or slow down your system, so be very clear on what your medication does so you know what to expect when you stop and how to deal with it.

As an overview, depression, whether it be major or minor, greatly changes our motivation. If you don't believe you can do it, or you don't believe you deserve to do it, you won't. This is why it is really important to address this issue, as it will make a massive difference to your results in not only managing your weight, but for everything else you want in your life.

This also why the *Rebel Diet* is designed the way it is. So that you can easily add it in and take it out when you want to; have a wonderful cheat day whilst still losing body fat; and there is no pressure or element of failure if you have a rough couple of days and fall off the wagon.

This is about creating freedom to be who you are and the person you want to be.

Time, family and the universe stop me!
How specifically do they stop you? What would happen if they didn't? What would you have to do, which you are not having to do now, if you did go ahead and start changing? What is the one thing you need to do in order to make time to do this, just for you?

Nothing really stops us from doing anything. I hear you raising your voice at me and flinging your arms about in dismay and irritation!

Let's put it this way, when it comes to changing your habits, it's more a question of getting used to a new routine. When you are dealing with work, family and all the other things that are sent to try us, usually there is a way around everything and frequently just talking it over with someone else can be very helpful as they may be more objective about being able to change your routine.

When we really want to or need to do something, usually we manage to make time to do it. The main objections we have about doing anything additional or different are usually due to being completely immersed in what is happening right now and it can be hard to see everything clearly.

Quite often it can feel like one big mess; in fact, by taking a step back for a moment and looking at ourselves and the responsibilities we feel we 'should' have, can help in re-evaluating our daily schedules and priorities.

This is another of the facets of the *Rebel Diet*. It's about creating time for you and making this for YOU.

Life can become a never-ending series of events for other people and sometimes it can feel like you have lost yourself. You don't know what you want any more, what clothes suit you any more, how your hair really suits. This is about taking back control and rediscovering YOU. It's about gaining motivation and self-belief at the same time as making the changes you want in your life.

> *'The only limit to our realization of tomorrow will be our doubts of today. Let us move forward with strong and active faith'*
>
> Franklin D Roosevelt

Chapter 4

Your Motivation (or lack of it)

Isn't it funny how you get all excited about doing something, get halfway through it and then all your drive disappears?

Maybe you find it really easy to help and support change in someone else – but find it difficult to do it for yourself? Or you are doing really well and then you have one little setback and everything just seems to stop?

You might identify with one of the above, or all three of them!?

There are lots of reasons why we lose or don't have motivation for creating change in ourselves.

This section is designed to explain some of the reasons why you may lose motivation so that you can address them, change them and make sure that you stay on track, fuelled with determination to make it work and keep it! It is actually a very big factor in why we succeed at anything, so this section doesn't just apply to this diet.

Secondary Gain

Now, this is something that I teach during our NLP courses. Secondary gain is where you gain something from doing or behaving in a certain way which is not advantageous to you. This also applies to weight loss. Of course, there are always people who don't have any secondary gain, but then they are usually the ones that can deal with the problem straight away so it doesn't recur.

As a therapist, before I get down to doing actual interventions, I always look for and deal with any reason, no matter how strange it might appear to be, why the person doesn't want to let go of the problem they are trying to change. This is the first thing I do with a client and we do not go forward until this is resolved.

When I say 'won't let go', what I mean is that the problem doesn't seem to be solved no matter what you do. You see, at some level, when you have a problem that you can't seem to resolve, there will be an underlying positive reason to have the problem which possibly at one time served a purpose, like protection or fear of failure, but now it is an unresourceful state and is not providing anything useful.

For example, one client who came to see me had terrible problems with always starting a diet and being really driven about it and then something would just almost switch off and she would stop. She would usually have lost about a stone in weight and then she said it was almost like a flick of a switch and she couldn't go on.

When we investigated her 'secondary gain', her reason to not let go of the problem, it turned out that every relationship which had failed she had blamed on her weight. Therefore, if she lost the weight and could no longer blame it on that, she would have to look at the real issues about why the relationship had failed. Not a pleasant thing to face and much easier to keep the weight on.

When we finally established the reason why the 'switch flicked off', she was able to deal with that issue and indeed went on to create the look she really wanted, unhindered. No more switch flicking!

Another example is someone who kept losing motivation as soon as she saw the diet starting to work. When we established the secondary gain, it seemed that the main area of concern was what she would 'have to do' once she lost weight, which was start to mix with people and socialise. This was a major problem for her, as her self-confidence was very low and the perception she had of herself was much worse than the reality.

So, by *not* losing weight, she wouldn't have to face those things she was most worried about and put herself in the uncomfortable position of 'being judged', which is what she believed would happen if she socialised or had to interact with people she didn't know.

Another common secondary gain is a fear of failure. Some people see themselves as a failure, so pushing something to 100% can be a very frightening place in case they do fail and therefore confirm to themselves they are a failure. It is must safer to quit or cause a problem, in which case they have to stop before taking it to a level where they could be deemed a success or a failure.

Very often, the secondary gain can seem silly to others but, if you think about it, there will be a very logical reason for it. Once you have identified the secondary gain, then you can really get started. Without establishing that, then you will be unlikely to make the changes that you want and this applies to almost anything.

Let's face it, if there was no secondary gain, you wouldn't have a problem, would you?

So, if you feel like something is stopping you, just like one of my clients, ask yourself 'What would I lose if I lost weight?' and 'What would change if I lost weight?' Are there any unresolved issues that are stopping you? Just remember, it may not appear to be logical, but these things are rarely logical on the surface. However, when you look at them objectively, you can understand why they are there and then solve them.

Ask yourself these questions and you can apply this to any problem you have that you find you can't change or resolve:

1) What positive thing will I gain if I solve this problem?
2) What positive thing will I lose if I solve this problem?
3) What will change if I solve this problem?
4) What will I have to do or deal with, which I am not currently having to do/deal with now, if I solve this problem?
5) What will happen if I don't solve this problem?
6) What won't happen if I don't solve this problem?

I know this looks simple, but you might be surprised at the answers you come up with which you may not have considered before. The key to this is not to think too hard about it and let the first thing which comes to mind leap out at you.

Towards or Away From?

Have you noticed how some things you desperately want you always seem to get while, with other things, you seem to get about halfway through and then lose motivation? This is what we call 'towards and away from' motivation.

Some people, when they decide to commit to doing something, are completely enthusiastic and work 'towards' what they want. The drive and desire to make that happen is really strong all the way through to completion, and they tend not to lose motivation as they progress towards what they DO want.

For instance, someone who is 'towards' and works in sales (hypothetically), is highly motivated by a really big bonus and will work towards that with 100% effort because that is what they want.

Also, someone who diets and perseveres until they reach the desired look and their motivation is unwavering throughout could be 'towards'. If they are also totally motivated by the vision in their head of how they *will* look and feel when they reach their goal, then that is really 'towards'.

Now, 'away from' is something really different

This means that your motivation comes from NOT WANTING or 'moving away from' something.

For instance, losing weight because you *don't* want to look the way you do any more, or trying to make more money because you don't want to be in a situation where you had no money in the past, are both examples of motivation by moving away from what you don't want.

The problem with 'away from' motivation is that when you get far enough away from what you don't want, then you feel it's safe to stop and the motivation drops.

So, you often only ever get 50 per cent to 80 per cent of what you wanted, which means you never get to where you want to be; you lose motivation as soon as you hit the 'safe' area, which is far enough away from the one thing that you desperately don't want.

So, going back to that hypothetical sales rep. If he was 'away from', then he would get no motivation at all from the big bonus he would get if he hit his sales target. His motivation would be that if he didn't hit his sales target he would get the sack, in which case he would work as hard as he could until he knew he was far enough 'away from' getting the sack, i.e. far enough away from what he doesn't want, then stops and never quite hits the target for the bonus.

The problem with 'away from' is that you never completely get to where you want to be. Like the sales rep. That is why a lot of us lose the motivation for something halfway through. If we can recognise it as it is happening, then we can change it and make sure we get exactly 100 per cent of what we want by focusing on what we want! I give the following true story as an example.

A lady I was working with came to me with a weight problem. She always promised herself she would look a certain way for a number of important occasions through her life, like her daughter's wedding, her son's graduation, or a presentation she had to give.

Every time she went on a diet, she always remembered how overweight she thought she had been and how much she disliked the way she looked. The motivation to lose the body fat was 'moving away' from what she didn't want.

So, she would motor off at 100 per cent and give the diet everything she had. Absolute determination to change, until she started to see results and then the motivation started to die away. The mental prison and restrictions on her for the diet she was using at the time took over; BUT she was far enough away from how she didn't want to look that she stopped dieting – but never really got to that image she had in her mind of how she really wanted to be.

So, when all of the 'towards and away from' was explained, she suddenly realised what she had been doing. We worked on what she really wanted and got her to keep that image of how she really wanted to look, which was that positive happy image and how she would feel when she got there.

This lady also did the *Rebel Diet* and, on her Rebel Days, made a pact with her husband that they would sit down together and work on their plan for their retirement and what they would do as well as raiding the local fish and chip shop!

Just that simple change made the difference between never achieving the image she had in her own mind and standing with her husband on their wedding anniversary party, looking just how she really wanted to.

A simple change in your own language and the way you think can drastically change your results.

When you focus on what you don't want to happen, then logically all your thoughts and determination go into that. So…what will you get? You will get what you don't want.

When you just change the thought process to thinking about what you *do* want and only concentrate on that one thing, your attitude and motivation changes; your entire drive and passion creates momentum and you make it happen.

A personal example is when I get nervous and start talking gibberish in front of someone I think is terribly important.

Ok, the best example I can think of is the day when I was training in the gym and Barry McGuigan had popped in to see Ricky Hatton (a world champion boxer) before a major televised fight which he was going to be commentating at. I assume you have worked out that I trained at the same gym Ricky trained at!

Anyway, my training partner knew that Barry McGuigan had been a long time hero of mine as he had battled his way to the top, had all the same crap I had from growing up and competing in Ireland and I had always wanted to meet him.

So, my training partner then disappeared and, unbeknown to me, had asked Barry to come and have a word with me. He had explained who I was, World Champion, etc., and that I had grown up in Belfast and was a big fan of his.

When I realised what had happened I had a fit of nerves and was trying to escape out of the door, just as I saw Mr McGuigan coming to greet me. Two people were holding the door shut so I couldn't get out and, when I fathomed there was no escaping, I made the fateful mistake of chanting to myself 'don't get nervous, don't talk gibberish' repeatedly in my head, nicely focusing on what I DIDN'T want to say to him.

So, as the poor man tried to make conversation, the most inane rubbish came out of my mouth and he must have thought I was a complete madwoman. If I had focused on being calm and asking him about his career then my anxiety would have lowered, my thoughts would have cleared and I could have had a meaningful couple of minutes with concise questions with an idol of mine, instead of a whirlwind of unrelated statements about the Bobby Sands hunger strike and the availability of clothing that fits an unusual shape! Hell, my stomach is tightening up as I write this.

The flip side of this, is when I was doing a TV programme which was presented by Donny Osmond. I was there as an expert contributor and, in between the actual shooting of the scenes, he wanted to talk to me about my competing and training. I completely focused on listening to him, taking my time in replying and being calm and, as a result, I had a very insightful conversation where I learnt a great deal about him and what he could bench press!

Moving swiftly on, that is a really small example of what a difference this can make.

These are pretty flippant examples of what I am trying to explain. However, if taken to even the deepest levels of what you want in your life and future, it can make a huge difference. It works with all of my clients, the people I coach and also in my own competing. Even telling an athlete before a 100m sprint international race, who had been focusing on not making the same mistakes again, to only think about what she wants to achieve and the feeling she will get from it, turned a badly performing runner into a Gold Medal sprinter that day.

Do this with something simple you have been tussling with for a while and you will see what I mean. The simple change of language in your own mind or even when you deal with other people can have some very impressive results.

Easier doing it for Others?
You may have found, possibly as you have got older, that the motivation for doing something for you is far less than doing it for someone else.

Being able to support, motivate and manoeuvre someone to lose weight is far easier than having the motivation for doing it for YOU.

As our life experiences and values change over the years, sometimes our own self-esteem becomes lower and our priority is no longer ourselves but our family and others we care about.

I have seen so many clients who tell me they don't really know who they are any more, they kind of got lost and life seems to be about everyone else. Taking time to do something on their own seems selfish and this is where I must differ.

Rebel Diet: Freeing You from Diet Hell

It is in fact more selfish not to take back 'you'

Of course, you will never forget about the other people in your life, but can you imagine how much happier everyone else around you would be if you were really happy and feeling good about yourself? Isn't it more selfish to deny those that love you the joy of seeing a happier and more confident person, who knows what they want and are comfortable with themselves?

Think about the last person you helped or saw blossom in front of your eyes – wasn't it wonderful? Well, turn that around now and think about how those that love you will feel if you take time for you, once a week, to do something you really want to do and REBEL, whilst changing how you look and feeling more comfortable with the skin you are in?

Just having one day a week, an hour even, just for you to rebel against a diet and everything else you want to fight against, makes a big difference.

Doing one small thing like this can change your outlook and, at the same time, change how others perceive you. What you project – for example, how you feel about everything and yourself, is projected out there.

Have you met people that you know deep down are unhappy? Do you remember how you felt when you were with someone like that and how you reacted to that person?

That is projection, and if you change your internal world to a happier place, then the outside world will be happier with you.

Sounds a bit strange doesn't it? Just try it and you will see what I mean!

> *'To know what you prefer instead of humbly saying Amen*
> *to what the world tells you you ought to prefer,*
> *is to have kept your soul alive'*
> Robert Louis Stevenson (1850-1894)

Chapter 5

Self Esteem, Mistakes and Faux pas

Life marches on and often we find ourselves millions of miles away from the days when a zit was disaster and a bad hair day meant meltdown.

Career, family, responsibilities and the needs of others begin to take hold and dominate our lives and time. You might be in that place right now and, if you are, you may also feel like you have lost 'you'.

It's almost like you don't know who you are any more, what clothes you like, your dreams and wants. This is about getting YOU back and this is also what your Rebel Day is all about.

When life revolves around everyone else and there seems to be no time left for you, your own confidence in yourself can lower. If you are also not happy about how you look this really does affect your self-esteem.

What I would love to be saying is that if you are not happy about your body image then don't worry, because this has no adverse reaction on any other area of your life. Unfortunately, it does.

Let's put it this way. If you are happy about how you look, then you feel confident and worry less about what others are thinking about you. This then increases your focus and is less distracting, your interaction with others is more confident and you have more natural rapport with other people.

As your self-esteem increases, as you grow more confident and you see your shape changing, notice how you feel in company and your interaction with others. This acts like a ripple effect through your life as you start to believe in your abilities and your outlook alters.

Simply by starting to do something for you once a week – your Rebel Day – will bring focus back to what you want and create a portal of time just for you.

I Just Lost It

We are all human. Things happen. Mistakes are made.

You may have been in a situation where you have been carefully following or doing something, then you make one mistake and that's it, finished and you can't go on.

You think 'I've blown it now, no point in trying to carry on...'

In a way, it's as though you were waiting for something to happen. You just knew it would anyway, you never succeed at anything so it was inevitable.

Does any of that sound familiar?

Sometimes, there can be a deep-seated belief in some people that they cannot succeed at anything they choose to do. That can either be a fear of pushing yourself to the crucial point where you find out if you succeed or fail, so you sabotage everything just before you get to that point; OR, you never even start, just in case you do fail and you confirm your worst fears.

You would be amazed at the number of people this applies to and, even more amazing, is the fact that they don't realise.

The difference with the *Rebel Diet* is that you can take a break, live your life, make a mistake and maybe fall off the wagon, but all you have to do is to pick up where you left off.

You see, when you know your diet routine for six days and then know you are having a major break day, a Rebel day, it makes it so much easier to feel like a success every week, building up your confidence continually.

Not only do we in fact FORCE you to have a cheat day, but if you fall off the wagon at any point – that's fine, so you don't feel like a failure. Because there is no failure.

Well that's not strictly true, as the only failure is believing you *are* a failure!

If you fall off the wagon, just get back on when you are ready because you have all the tools to carry on. With this system, it's about using it when you want to and knowing which diet to use and when.

Fear of Failure

For a lot of us, when we feel we have failed at something, the hardest part is rectifying it. When we rectify something, it means having to face what we believe we have failed at.

Now, just stop and take a minute to think about this. How many people have you heard talking about doing things and never do them? Loads of them I bet!

So – if you have actually started something and are doing it, even if you make a mistake, do you really 'fail' if you make that mistake? Compare yourself to all those people who say they will do things and never do.

Can you think of something you did, made a mistake, learned from it and then when you tried it again you were so much better because you learned something from it? Would you have called that a failure? No, you wouldn't!

If something doesn't work for you, then, as long as you learn from it, you can use those learnings to make it succeed next time and give you a better understanding. Or, make many mistakes and become a complete expert and write a book about it!

So, mistakes sometimes need to be made in order to do something really well or move to the next level and be able to perfect what you are doing.

Now, without wanting to sound too 'muesli and crystals', learning from a past event, situation or any other occurrence helps you to separate negative emotions associated with that event and assists you in moving on to be even better.

You then begin to associate what you originally perceived as 'failure' as a positive learning experience (maybe after a bit of wailing and gnashing of teeth!); this then becomes a learned behaviour and any fear of failure begins to disappear and really starts helping you get what you WANT and believe you can DAMN WELL GET IT!

As I mentioned earlier, there can sometimes be a deep-seated belief in certain people that they cannot succeed at anything they choose to do. This tends to only be in one area of their life. Most people don't believe that absolutely everything they do will end in mayhem, it's usually just one part of their life (if they did, they probably wouldn't bother getting out of bed!).

For instance, I have worked with many very successful business people, actors, entrepreneurs, athletes and, heaven forbid, writers. Now, they knew they could succeed in that part of their life, but when it came to something in their personal life which was just for them, that's when the doubt crept in.

Like a silent Stepford wife invasion, the doubt eased its way in, infiltrated and then multiplied to cause total doubt in their ability to do anything about their weight.

Now, the actual fear of failure is pretty straightforward. That can either be:

1) A fear of pushing yourself to the point where you have to give it 100 per cent. You are worried about not succeeding because, if you don't succeed, then you are confirming your worst fears that you are a failure. A special feature of this issue is always managing to create a crisis or problem so that you never have to take it to 100 per cent.

2) A belief that you will fail – which means you are doomed before you even start!

This is a self-confidence problem which you can deal with by taking each day as it comes. You notice how good you feel each day you succeed and congratulate yourself at the end of each successful day. That way it doesn't seem like such a mammoth haul (as you know, it isn't a mammoth haul, it's just that with this problem it usually feels like it is!).

So, if you find that you do fall off this diet for whatever reason, then see what happened to cause you to cheat. Adjust and learn from it and start again – next time you will have the extra knowledge and can do it even better!

One of the great things about this *Rebel Diet* is that once a week you can take a break, rebel, eat whatever you want, speed your metabolism up and then start again.

You don't see endless days of dieting, just six

Then you can enjoy eating cream cakes and whatever you want on the seventh day! So the benefit is twofold: it gives you a break and gives your metabolism a kick!

'If you have made mistakes, even serious ones,
there is always another chance for you.
What we call failure is not the falling down
But the staying down'

Mary Pickford (1893-1979)

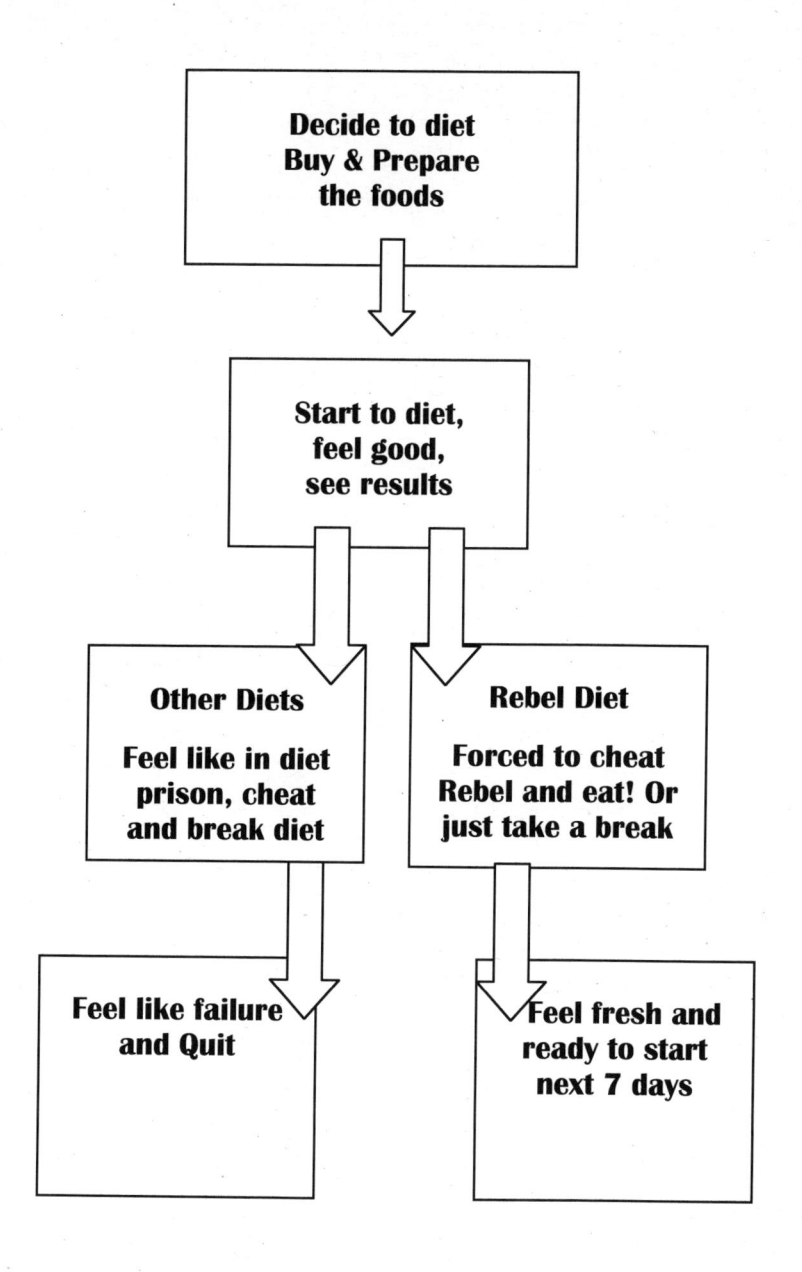

Rebel Diet: Freeing You from Diet Hell

```
┌─────────────────────┐
│   Decide to diet    │
│   Buy & Prepare     │
│     the foods       │
└──────────┬──────────┘
           ▼
┌─────────────────────┐
│    Start to diet,   │
│     feel good,      │
│    see results      │
└─────┬─────────┬─────┘
      ▼         ▼
┌───────────┐ ┌───────────┐
│Other Diets│ │Rebel Diet │
│           │ │           │
│Feel like  │ │Forced to  │
│in diet    │ │cheat      │
│prison,    │ │Rebel and  │
│cheat and  │ │eat! Or    │
│break diet │ │just take  │
│           │ │a break    │
└─────┬─────┘ └─────┬─────┘
      ▼             ▼
┌───────────┐ ┌───────────┐
│Feel like  │ │Feel fresh │
│failure    │ │and ready  │
│and Quit   │ │to start   │
│           │ │next 7 days│
└───────────┘ └───────────┘
```

Chapter 6

Body Image & The 3 Me's

Body image – how we see ourselves in our own mind's eye and what we see in the mirror – is the biggest motivating factor to change our body shape. What we see and how we view it can be considerably different to reality.

You may not be comfortable with what you see in the mirror, or with what you believe other people see when they look at you. However, you may be comfortable with yourself and how you see yourself, but when you are in public you become self-conscious about your appearance.

When I am working with a client who has body dysmorphic disorder (severe self-image distortion), I always find out how they see themselves in three different ways. For more information on body dysmorphic disorder, please see my therapy site www.emmajames.net.

Each perspective is usually different and gives an indicator as to where the problem lies. The three me's – or how you see yourself in three different spheres – are:

1) What you think you look like when you think about yourself.
2) How you think family or close friends see you when they look at you.
3) How you think strangers who have never met you before see you.

Close your eyes and think of each one. Do you have a picture? When you do, do you notice how you look in each one? Do you notice if you look distorted in all or any of them? If you do, is that situation one that you feel uncomfortable in?

This is a huge insight into where your insecurities lie and whether in fact you have a distorted body image.

Some people will have an accurate view of how they look in their own mind and when they are with friends and family. However, when asked how they believe they look in the third picture, to a group of people they have never met before, then the description begins to change to a less favourable one.

I can tell you from a personal perspective that when I had exercise anorexia, the three me's were significantly different. The 'me' I saw of myself in my head was fat with bulging areas of fat at my hips, lower abdominal area, lower back and my face looked like a chipmunk.

The picture I saw of myself in front of family and friends was facially grotesque with the same body.

What I believed strangers saw when they looked at me was a woman akin to a beached whale with no physique. So, my interaction at the time with people I didn't know was pretty shocking, and I avoided social situations and outings to places like shopping centres like the plague.

Competing was fine, because this was my 'confident' self, one area in my life where I had a lot of experience and felt self-assured. Plus, I also knew the ropes and this was my 'comfort zone'.

That is a pretty extreme example, but what is important is that if your self body image is distorted negatively, you need to be aware of that and notice how it changes as your confidence grows.

During the times when I was competing or training, what I saw in the mirror was always considerably better than at times when I felt low or vulnerable.

My clients have the same situations and this is what I look for, as they really do give you insight into what areas of their lives need to change and how in fact they view themselves.

Bad Hair Days

Our own self-image changes according to the frame of mind we are in. Most people will have a degree of distortion in their body image, especially if they are having a 'bad hair day'. Now this doesn't mean that you have any issues as such, it can be just a simple off day.

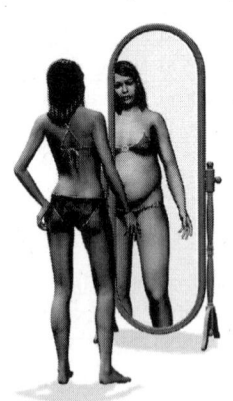

What we imagine we look like and what we see in the mirror is very much dependant on how we are feeling at the time. When you have a good day you tend to feel more confident and therefore feel better about yourself – this will also affect the perception of yourself and how you think other people see you.

This is the same for when you are not happy. If you are depressed or have a low self-esteem, the likelihood is that you may have a distorted self body image and the picture you see is one that is in fact worse than in reality.

Being around people when your body image is distorted can be uncomfortable and difficult and can lead to a reluctance to go out in public, eating disorders, further lack of self confidence etc.

If you find that your own self-image varies considerably depending on your mood, then you need to be very sure that you do in fact need to lose weight. A big clue may be when people tell you not to lose any more or being genuinely surprised when you state you want to lose weight. If that happens, rather than believing everyone are idiots, ask yourself if your own body image is distorted.

If you do have the weight to lose and your body image is somewhat distorted, then you will notice a difference in your own self-confidence as your self-image improves on a daily basis.

If you do happen to get up one morning and you don't like what you see – think about what is happening in your life and how that may be affecting what you see through your moods.

Remember, if you are a woman coming up to you period, there is a hormonal shift. This not only means that there may be a noticeable mood swing and therefore an effect on you self body image, but also considerable water retention, which will make you feel bloated and will possibly affect how you feel in your clothes. However, this is only temporary and will normally rectify itself within a few days.

Any men out there reading this, I can tell you that this is a very good piece of information which could score you major brownie points if you happen to mention that your female partner looks wonderful when you know she is feeling pretty low and pre-menstrual!

Remember, if you are in a negative frame of mind and have a distorted image of yourself, then it is harder to motivate yourself to change. Again, this is where concentrating on your Rebel Day makes a difference.

Doing something special just for you is your reward for the work you have put in during the six days, creates positive momentum and starts to shift the negative mindset. You can eat VERY naughty stuff with the knowledge it is in fact speeding up your metabolism! How perfect is that?!

The Jaffa Cake invasion!
Yes, that's right - Jaffa cakes.

I have been known to comfort eat on occasions, but luckily this was something which I could control.

Comfort eating, bingeing and compulsive overeating are all things which have become more prevalent in our society today. Whether this is because their frequency has actually increased or because they are given more publicity and are therefore less of a taboo, we are not certain. Either way, more people are seeking assistance for these conditions than ever before.

This section is for those of you, and I know you are out there, who are sufferers. For binge eating, compulsive overeating and bulimia, it is always advisable to seek therapeutic or medical help, but here is some information which you might find useful from my own treatment of these conditions with my clients.

Obviously, if this doesn't apply to you then you may as well skip onto the next chapter!

Comfort Eating

Many people deal with a comfort eating issue. Some find it only happens occasionally and they 'allow' themselves to do it, thus making it a controlled decision and with little or no adverse effect.

However, for others, it is a repetitive behaviour which can feel embarrassing and can also bring with it feelings of self-loathing and guilt, which certainly then has a continuing negative influence on your self-esteem and belief in your ability to succeed.

So, then, what is comfort eating? Well, it is generally perceived as some kind of greed or food related issue.

I can tell you now that this is absolutely not the case and woe betide anyone who says that in front of me!

Comfort eating is simply a learned behaviour where the brain has associated a way of getting back some kind of comfort through food. This happens when we are feeling a certain way, for instance when we are feeling low, bored, stressed etc. Then the learned behaviour kicks in in order to make us feel the way we want to feel – for example, better or comforted.

So, frequently we will have a particular type of food which is a comforter. For me it is Jaffa cakes, for some it is boiled sweets, for others it's crisps or a thousand different things.

The learned behaviour will have happened at some point in your life where you felt better or felt excited in relation to food. This is a neurological connection which has been made. So, when the chain reaction starts, e.g. you feel stressed, the chain starts and the cravings for sweets kick in; you feel a genuine need, you eat, feel temporarily better and then the guilt begins with all the negative emotion attached.

To give you an example, a client of mine came to see me with a comfort eating issue. We took it right back to the emotion she felt just before she would get the craving or the need to eat. For her, it was when she felt lonely. Normally this would happen when she was at home on her own and she would be sitting on the settee watching television. She always sat on the end seat of the settee, as this was the best view for the television.

She would get the feeling of loneliness, then get the craving for bags of sweets, like toffees etc.

I asked her what did she feel when she started to eat, right at the start. What was the very first feeling she would get when she put that first sweet in her mouth? She stated it was a feeling of being secure, loved and calm.

The next stage was to identify a time when she felt this way and was eating sweets and she said straight away that it was when she was a child. Her Father would work away from home all week and come back every Friday night. Her Mother would then go out to take her sister to a ballet lesson, leaving her with her Father. She would sit on her Father's knee, just the two of them on the end of the settee, as this was the best place to sit to watch the television. They would then eat sweets he had brought back for the two of them. They were some of the happiest memories she had with her Father. So:

1) We identified the trigger, for example the emotion she felt that started the whole cycle, which was loneliness.
2) The way she wanted to feel was loved and secure, so the learned behaviour which was ingrained was to do something to feel that way.
3) The way to get that back was to recreate an association with something which gave her that feeling again.
4) We then had the reason for the comfort eating and the strategy which triggered the entire behaviour.

At that point I did a number of NLP techniques with her, which then stopped the entire behaviour.

Here is something simple you can do to combat the behaviour yourself. Remember – this is only if it isn't severe and sometimes you will need outside assistance if the problem is complex and has other issues attached.

You are quite simply going to use what we call a 'pattern Interrupt'. This is just a way of interrupting a pattern of behaviour which then causes it to falter and then stop. The major key with this is to be able to send the behaviour in a new direction and away from what you had been previously doing.

- First, identify the feeling you have just before the feeling of needing to eat. This will be a negative emotion, like boredom, stress, a certain low feeling etc
- Second, be aware that once you feel that emotion, the next stage

may be a craving and a feeling of needing to eat
- Third, decide on something you can do at any time when you get that negative emotion BEFORE you feel you need to eat. It could be to call someone, take the dog for a walk, write a list of goals you want to achieve. You could also think of other things which give you a feeling of happiness, confidence, or a feeling of achievement once you have done them. Only you will know what they are

This simple series of steps stops the craving for comfort eating from ever starting; in fact, it begins another learned behaviour which, over time and if continually repeated, will become ingrained.

By the way, the client I was telling you about simply stopped comfort eating and lost two and a half stone. We deliberately didn't implement a diet, we just wanted to see how much weight she would lose without altering her diet. She is a real superstar though, as all my clients are!

Binge Eating Disorder (BED)

Binge Eating Disorder has only recently been recognised as a condition in its own right. The reason for this was that a clear defining line between bulimia and binge eating needed to be made. Obviously, binge eating happens in varying degrees but the main difference between binge eating and bulimia is that people suffering from BED do not purge (make themselves sick) after bingeing.

It is believed that many more people suffer from binge eating disorder than either anorexia or bulimia. The problem is that, because of the amount of food eaten, many people with BED become obese and this can lead to problems with blood pressure, heart disease and can also have an adverse effect on their mental state.

The treatment for BED is in some ways similar to that for bulimia and you would be urged to seek assistance with this.

Binge eating is very different from comfort eating because the cravings are so severe and intense that it is completely overwhelming. If you have never experienced it, then I don't think I could put it into words for you to understand. Those of you who do know what it is like, then you may be nodding your head when you think back to the times when you have tried to explain the feeling.

Normally, when I deal with BED, we start off with interrupting the pattern of the bingeing before altering anything else in the diet. Once that has settled then we would begin to work on the dieting. Usually a significant amount of weight has been lost by then and we know where we are with the metabolism.

If you *do* suffer with BED and would like to use the strategy outlined for the Comfort Eating, then you might find it could help, although I would still advise seeing a professional.

Another point to make is that with long term binge eating, bulimia, anorexia and any other serious eating disorder, once removed, there is in fact a bereavement period. Remember, this process has taken up a lot of time and thought process and usually filled a part of that person's day for a very long time.

Getting used to being without it and, in a way, grieving, is quite normal but is also the most turbulent time for the sufferer.

Signs of binge eating:

1) Intense craving and physical need to eat.
2) A feeling of anticipation or build-up before a binge or during the planning of it.
3) Eating much more quickly than usual.
4) Eating until feeling uncomfortably full.
5) Eating large amounts of food when not actually hungry.
6) Eating alone or hiding food because of embarrassment at the amounts of food consumed.
7) Feeling out of control around food.
8) Feeling very self-conscious eating in front of others in case you are judged.
9) Feeling shameful, depressed or guilty after bingeing.
10) Being unable to purge or compensate for the food eaten.

One client who I treated for a binge eating disorder, whose trigger was a feeling of being 'low' in a specific way which would have sent him to find any savoury foods like crisps and sandwiches, walks past the fridge in the kitchen to the cupboard beside it and gets out a pack of cards and plays cards with his partner.

It's simple to treat, but breaking down the actual step-by-step strategy can take a little time.

Compulsive Overeating

Compulsive Overeating is a variation on binge eating, but you will eat at times when you are not hungry. This may happen all the time or it may come and go in cycles.

Most people who are compulsive eaters are overweight, and may use their weight or appearance as a shield they can hide behind to avoid social interaction; others hide behind a happy or jolly façade to avoid confronting their problems. Sufferers often have great shame at being unable to control the compulsion to eat. Compulsive overeating is a serious condition and needs professional support to ensure long term recovery.

This normally will be a mix of quite severe low self-esteem and confidence along with a strategy or pattern of behaviour that makes them feel better when they get quite low or unhappy/stressed. Again, it is a matter of finding a pattern interrupt, but also working on the self-esteem issues and assisting that person in really gaining confidence in themselves and who they are - plus where they want to be.

Overall
Any kind of eating issue or disorder is generally embarrassing to discuss and deal with. It is one of the hardest issues to openly divulge, which is incredible seeing as such emphasis is placed on the social importance of eating and cooking AND the amount of cooking programmes on television!

However, there is support and therapy available and, believe me, you are NOT alone. This is a treatable issue as so many people have found out and that includes me as well!

> *'We did not change as we grew older;*
> *we just became more clearly ourselves'*
> Lynn Hall, *Where Have All the Tigers Gone? (1989)*

Chapter 7

Metabolic Monster

Why does the Rebel Diet work?
Well, the basis of the entire physical diet is your metabolic rate. And no, this isn't another metabolic diet!

Your metabolism is how the fuel (food) is broken down in your system and how the components are then transported to the rest of your body where they are needed.

There are *varying speeds* your metabolism will work at and this will determine if you are:

- Thin and able to eat anything you want (grrrrrrr!)
- Someone who easily maintains a weight they are happy with, or
- Constantly battling against putting on body fat and fighting to keep it off

Now, this is where it all gets interesting. The slower the metabolic rate, the slower you burn your fuel. This means that any excess which isn't burnt off goes into storage in preparation for a long term famine or a sudden need to use all that stored fuel for a sudden major trauma. Very efficient really, although a bit melodramatic!!

The Rebel Diet has come from my own battle with having a slow metabolism and needing to keep my weight down for competing, plus self-confidence and a bit of vanity thrown in.

It has also grown and developed from working with others over the years and learning how their bodies react to various strategies. Through this I have been able to find the common factors which work for those of us afflicted with a stubborn weight issue.

One of the other things I have done over the years is to deal with a number of female athletes who, because of their sport, have needed to get down to 5 per cent body fat. I can tell you that this is where all the techniques found have been proven over and over again.

With my own therapy clients, from working with stress, anxiety and varying other issues over the years, ultimately we have had to look at the other problems which have had an effect on the metabolism and deal with those in conjunction with the physical methods of raising the metabolism through diet, exercise etc.

Through all of this, I have had to learn the tricks which do work, don't work, are plain old wives' tales OR just simply dangerous.

One of the MAJOR factors of this diet is that you are in fact *forced to have a cheat day! An eat anything you want day. A live your life to the full day.*

What is Metabolism?

It's the amount of energy (calories) your body burns to maintain itself. Metabolism is the process by which nutrients are acquired, transported, used and disposed of by the body. Quite simply, the broken down content of what you eat.

It is like a conveyor-belt process and it's this process of the breakdown and feeding of the rest of the body with those essential components which is the 'metabolism'.

Everyone has a different metabolism that will be unique to them. The metabolism is simply the process of using the energy and having its components carted off to the right places for use. Sometimes an imbalance can occur in the level of what is used after it has been broken down and transported, meaning that there is a residue left unused and this is what is then stored as body fat.

You can also go the other way completely, where the process happens so fast that the body starts using the tissue and muscle as fuel because it has used up everything you have put in. In this situation you end up very thin!

If someone who normally is relatively sedentary throughout the day is consuming far too much 'energy' then there will be an excess amount which will be whipped off to the fat stores. If that person begins an exercise routine while still consuming the same amount of 'energy', then the demand will change and more, if not all, of the excess energy will be effectively used by the body rather than going for storage.

Your metabolism is the major key to this whole situation of getting stubborn weight off. Don't think of it like 'just a process'; it's almost like another personality with a mind of its own which acts and reacts in certain ways, all of them very individual. And one of the ways of changing that is by changing the demand.

Within the metabolism process there are two basic functions that happen when the fuel is broken down.

1) Anabolism

It is simply a building process. Elements of the fuel are taken away and transported to places they are needed for building, e.g. muscle tissue, immune system etc.

2) Catabolism

The breaking down phase of metabolism, the opposite of anabolism. Catabolism includes all the processes by which complex substances are progressively broken down into simpler ones and then utilised by the body.

Your metabolism works at varying speeds, depending on many different external and internal factors. The speed at which it works is termed your 'Metabolic Rate'.

You can generally feel when your metabolism has increased. You feel the warmth of the rate increasing; you feel like you have more energy and are more alert. In fact, you would feel as though you had taken some kind of mild stimulant. It is quite amazing when you feel it.

Emma James

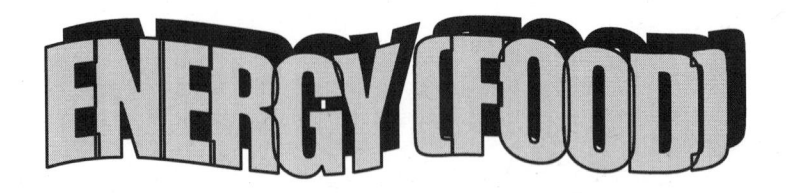

ENERGY (FOOD)

DIGESTED

Muscles
Connective tissue
Brain
Bone

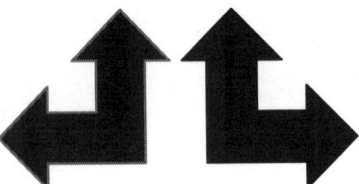

Blood
VitalOrgans
Bone

Energy Storage

Transported to various parts of the body

Your Metabolic Rate
This is the rate at which your body uses the fuel you have put into it. It is also a very good indication as to how to deal with the weight issue you have and to what is going on at the moment.

Depending on the answers you have given regarding your current situation and lifestyle, you have probably established the speed at which your metabolic rate is currently working. It may be a bit slow, very slow or almost completely ground to a halt!

Now, we can move on to what to do with you!

Just remember, that putting on weight or finding it hard to lose weight can sometimes be due to a medical condition so make sure you see your GP and get the 'all clear' before you start.

The two metabolic rates which usually cause some problems are the fast and the slow ones. People who complain of not being able to put on weight and those who complain of not being able to lose it!

So what exactly is the metabolic rate?
As you know by now, the metabolic rate is the rate at which the body burns fuel. It goes into your body and gets transported into the stomach, where it is broken down into its useful components and whipped off for use throughout the body.

The bits that are left over and not utilised are then stored, as there is nowhere for them to go. They are stored as body fat at this point and each person will have a natural disposition to store fat in certain places. Again, this is an individual thing. HOWEVER, on a very general basis, men tend to hold body fat on their stomachs and lower back and women tend to store it on the top of the thighs, the hips, bottom, lower abdominal area (although this is frequently water retention) and arms.

Now then, this is where is starts getting tricky.

If you have a slow metabolic rate the speed at which fuel is burnt is generally pretty sluggish, so there is more excess before the next load is put in and therefore you will store more fat.

Now – the whole aim of this diet system is to learn how to:

- Keep your metabolic rate raised
- Recognise when it is slowing down
- Have the knowledge of what to do to speed it up

This is where the rebel days come in as a REALLY important part of the entire process. To hell with chemicals, starvation and lettuce diets – let's get your metabolism moving, be able to eat and be able to have a life and take control of your body.

One of the major fallacies of dieting is that you have to decrease what you are eating. Absolute balderdash.

To lose body fat – you must eat.

The most common complaint is 'But I only eat once a day and I put weight on'. Well, of course you do! If I was your body and got rationed with only one meal a day I would slow down to a really slow rate and store every morsel you gave me! It's logical, so everything that gets put in is stored.

Obviously there are extremes to this. For instance anorexia – for most anorexics, their bodies' metabolic rate has slowed down so much they can in fact survive on tiny amounts of food because their metabolism has virtually stopped to keep them alive.

That is a very simplistic explanation though.

STRESS   **NOT EATING MUCH**   **TRAUMA**
DEPRESSION
TOO LITTLE CARBOHYDRATE

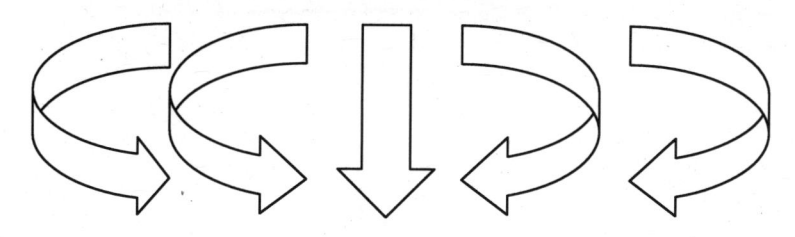

Body thinks it is under attack
Must conserve energy and preserve the body

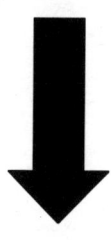

SLOWS METABOLISM TO PROTECT THE BODY

'The meeting of two personalities is like the contact of two chemical substances: if there is any reaction, both are transformed'
Carl Jung (1875-1961)

Chapter 8

The Knicker Effect

Repeated Dieting and The Effect On Your Metabolism
Why the 'Knicker Effect'? Well, did you ever hear the saying 'up and down like a lady of the night's knickers'?

This is the same as repeated or yo-yo dieting. Weight going up and down constantly!

If you are among those who have been searching for 'the answer' for a long time then you may have been dieting for what seems an eternity.

You could be going from one diet to another, gaining and losing weight, staying on some for a while and staying on others for a few days. The problem with this is that even if you have had a normal metabolic rate prior to lengthy dieting, you may in fact have slowed it down considerably through 'knicker effect' dieting.

This is a common problem, and if you can raise your hand to the following questions then you have probably slowed your metabolic rate considerably.

Have you:

1) After another diet, come off and then put more weight on than you lost?
2) Gone back to a normal healthy diet which in fact shouldn't precipitate weight gain but, for some reason, you put it on?
3) Always have initial short success and then the progress just seems to stop?
4) Really push the dieting and find that you just can't lose weight the way you expect to, even if you exercise?

If you answer yes to any of those questions then you are probably suffering from your metabolism slowing due to repeated dieting.

What happens is that the body thinks that it is being continually starved and therefore slows down so that it will conserve all the stores needed for the famine that it appears to be having!

It also seems that the body gets quite adept at working out what you are doing and slowing down just to put a spanner in the works! Although this isn't really the case, it certainly seems like it sometimes.

Let's put it into another context.

When a bodybuilder, who has to reduce his body fat down to 4% or 5%, finishes competing after an intensive 16 week diet, great effort is need to make sure that the metabolism stays raised to ensure continued fat loss. The metabolism will certainly have slowed to a degree as the body fat is now down to unnaturally and unhealthily low levels. The athlete then has to go 'off season' and really pour the calories in; otherwise, the next time he diets down for competition, the diet will not work to the same degree as before.

The purpose of explaining all this will become clear in a moment.

A boxer has trained hard and has had to lose up to 4 or 5 kilos of body fat to make his weight category and then fight - he has to go 'off season' as well and eat, put weight back on and get his metabolic rate back up to 'normal operating levels'. In this way, the next time he needs to drop the weight, he can diet down quickly and easily. He has to increase his food intake, calories, fats etc., to get the body to restore itself back to the normal metabolic rate it was at before he started dieting.

Unfortunately, due to the press not having a clue about 'off season' and sports nutrition, these athletes then have unkind things printed about them in the press. One particular boxer springs to mind who experiences this every time.

If they don't do this, then their metabolism will remain slower and it will be very difficult or impossible to get the body fat levels down to the same degree next time they compete as the diet just wont be as effective.

These are quite extreme examples, as you won't be swing dieting like that, but they do illustrate the point that you MUST take time out from dieting to FORCE the metabolism to speed up.

So, in other words, to make a diet work and maintain the weight you want, you MUST have break days to make sure the body restores itself back to its normal rate.

Sometimes, a person has been dieting for so long that a different approach has to be taken – again they are FORCED TO REBEL against all the previous diet industry twaddle and actually eat foods which would normally not be allowed – like junk food and bread - for a week to really push the metabolism and force it to speed up. I will show you how to do this later.

The Mental Drawbacks of the Knicker Effect

The mental side effect of yo-yo dieting is that your self-confidence in your ability tends to become lower at this point in time due to repeated attempts to diet and not getting the results that you want.

Then your motivation frequently becomes lower as you think 'What's the point?' as nothing seems to work the way you want, and your self-image can also suffer.

Belief in 'you' and what you are doing is really important as well.

It's sometimes difficult to completely believe that you can achieve something – and you know what, that's ok. Repeated dieting can really begin to knock your confidence. As your metabolism continually slows down from having to leap into survival mode, you can start to lose belief in yourself.

Small, yet sustained, achievable steps with no pressure gradually build up that self belief again.

I remember getting ready for a competition and I was over the weight limit. As I mentioned, I have a predisposition to putting weight on so this is not an unknown situation! I was in panic mode as usual, stressed and working REALLY hard at losing the body weight. Now, remember that everything in the mind will affect the body – the reactions and abreactions. So, of course, my metabolism went into slow down and survival mode and I had real trouble in losing the weight.

However, the second I decided, 'Sod it, I'll just have to go up a weight category,' then the weight began to come off. This was one of the first realisations at that time about mental state and physical reaction.

Now, during that stressed time of TRYING REALLY HARD to lose the body weight, I had lost confidence in myself which was also affecting my training and my results. It was affecting my studies as well. It just seemed to seep into every area of my life.

When I made that decision to go into the next weight category with the 'big birds' and to hell with it, my disposition changed. As a result of this change of attitude:

1) My training improved again and I was on target.
2) I noticed that my weight had begun to drop.
3) I felt better about myself.
4) I didn't feel such a failure. I started to take each step of dieting down without the pressure that I had before. I made weight and took the title!

Now this occurrence was at a time when I had been continually dieting on and off. Each time I was trying to drop the weight before a competition I was finding it harder than the previous time.

I was also not really coming off my diet in-between competitions so, unbeknown to me, my system was getting slower and slower all the time as it constantly thought it was under attack by not being given enough energy (carbohydrate) to meet the demands I was putting on myself.

At that time it was not common knowledge that you had to go 'off season' and allow your body to normalise again so that, when you needed to drop weight again, the metabolism would allow it to happen instead of being in a state of resistance when you needed it to comply the most.

This was the beginning of the understanding about the relationship between the brain, the emotional state and what will hinder and help in the fight to maintain a bodyweight and/or shape you are happy with.

Of course, most people thought I was mad. Amongst my peers, who were mostly men, many of them didn't have this problem and also hadn't been continually dieting on and off for any length of time.

It wasn't understood how repeated dieting could affect your metabolic rate and how it caused it to slow down and become resistant. Now, it is a researched and known fact and one of the key factors in the work I do with clients and how I get it revved up again and working.

Remember, the stress of yo-yo dieting as well as the chemical reactions it creates in the brain will send signals to the body to get into 'survival' mode again. It's like one big continual stress and assault on the mind and body, so no wonder that for some it results in a protection mode to keep them safe. How sensible is that?! Infuriating, but sensible!

Remember that you will learn how to monitor, regulate and change your own metabolism through the programme here, so don't panic!

Lifestyle and Adrenal Burnout
Being able to structure life, family, work and all the things that get in the way can be a wee bit tricky!!

However, the more stress you can take out of your life, the better your system will work. The thing is that if you are under stress a lot of the time a couple of things may happen.

Your adrenaline production increases – now if your adrenaline production is raised for a long period time it can cause something called *adrenal burnout*.

I could get all technical here but it wouldn't really serve any purpose!

Adrenal burnout
If you are pumping out adrenaline with your body in a state of stress over a long time your body thinks to itself 'Blimey, I'm under some serious threat here' and so does the sensible thing and slows everything down, so as to preserve the body in its time of 'trauma'.

A very sensible thing too!!

However, if it is a long term situation or there are a succession of events which you get stressed about, then it means that your system is running in 'Help, I'm being attacked' mode for a long time and it almost becomes normal for it to run at that speed.

So – doing anything that will combat that stress, or at least assist in combating it, is a huge step forward to getting your system back up to speed. This is where the Rebel Diet comes in. The non-pressure, easy structure and the benefit of the REBEL DAY, where you must do something for yourself, begins to take the edge off and allows your system to wind down slightly each time you do it.

We could at this stage go into cortisol production and body fat retention but that is probably for another time!

Being able to take a step back from each situation and take a view as though you are watching yourself in a movie can help get each event into perspective. I'm not saying it is a 'cure all' but by just running the situation in your head can sometimes help regain a feeling of control and a clearer view of what is going on.

Time management can also cause a lot of stress

What or who can you kick into touch and reorganise?

Who is it you running after who, in fact, could be looking after themselves? How can you steal that sacred 20 minutes of 'my time', even if it is locked in the loo away from everyone?

Just changing a few things in your day can make a huge difference and help make things feel a bit less stressed.

Finally – your rebel day. This isn't just a cheat day

This is YOUR day. Your day, to do what you want. It is not only about total freedom to eat what you want, but also to do something new and start the changes in your life as well as your body.

It could be something outrageous, it could be something challenging or silly or anything you want, BUT it MUST be for you.

This is really important – *to get to where you want to be* you have to be worth it. If you don't think you are worth it, then you will never get where you want to be. If you rebel, you must think – deep down, at some level – you are worth it.

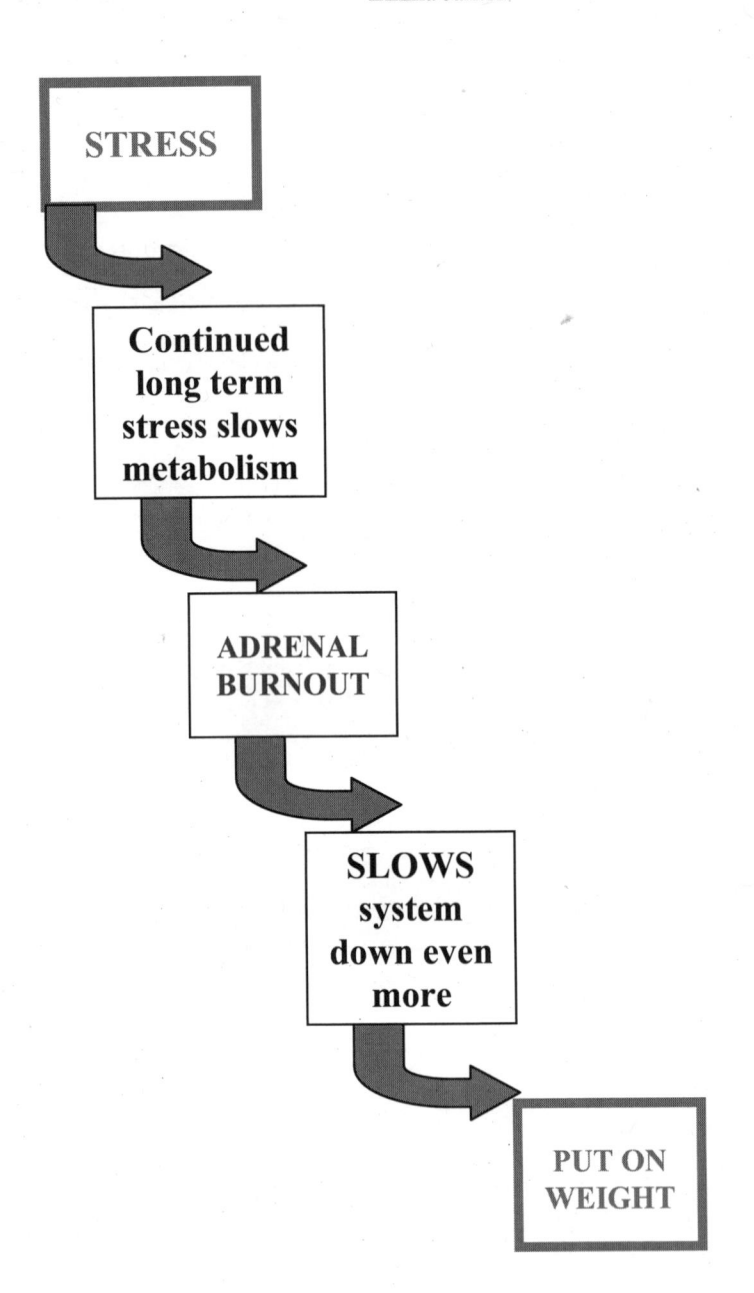

```
STRESS
   ↓
Continued long term stress slows metabolism
   ↓
ADRENAL BURNOUT
   ↓
SLOWS system down even more
   ↓
PUT ON WEIGHT
```

Chapter 9

Fast & Slow Metabolic Rates

Fast Metabolic Rate
Now, I do realise that having a section about fast metabolic rates in this book is possibly nonsensical. However, it's pretty good to know a little bit about the fast metabolic rate.

It also helps, when you feel like chopping someone into tiny pieces because they eat everything and anything they want, just to recognise that they simply have a faster metabolic rate.

A person with a fast metabolism will generally have the following characteristics:

1) Generally be thin or carrying little body fat.
2) Have high energy levels and/or be very active.
3) Be able to consume foods containing high fats and sugars consistently and put on little body fat.
4) Find it difficult to put on muscle mass.
5) Find it difficult to put on any weight including fat.

People with a fast metabolic rate may also complain of being hungry frequently and become hypoglycaemic if they don't eat frequently. As the fuel that is put into their system is being burnt so quickly, they need to 'refuel' frequently.

Of course, you may recognise this in quite a few gangly teenagers who spend their time trying to work out how on earth to get weight on and who have pictures of Arnie on their walls.

Anyone with a highly active routine, who trains heavily, or generally exerts high levels of energy throughout the day, may not in fact have a high metabolic rate. They may have a pretty stable rate which has been elevated by a high energy demand.

There could be any number of factors which will cause them to have difficulty putting and keeping weight on.

When presented with someone who has this issue, the first thing I have to work out is if they have got a naturally fast metabolic rate. Then I need to look at lifestyle factors which will add to the problem and discover if there is anything which could be altered or changed to allow the system to slow down.

For instance:

1) If they have a medical condition – they will have been to see their GP for a health screen before they come to see me.
2) Lifestyle pace.
3) Stress (if they react to general stress with the metabolic rate consistently staying high).
4) If they train and to what level – then look at the diet to see if they are burning off more fuel than is being put in.
5) How much muscle mass they have, as this also increases metabolic rate.

So, you see, there are lots of pitfalls for the gangly people of our world; so don't be too harsh on them, even though it is tempting to hang them out of a window!

NOTE. Those of you with a high metabolic rate should see your GP for a full health screen and thyroid and blood sugar tests before using any diet format.

Slow Metabolic Rate

A person with a slow metabolic rate will generally present some of the following characteristics:

1) Excess body fat.
2) Find it difficult to keep body fat levels down.
3) Feel tired.
4) Put body fat on easily even with a balanced diet.
5) May put muscle mass on easily.
6) Eat infrequently and still put on weight.

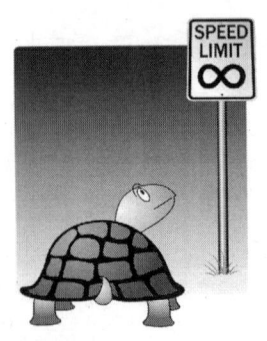

When the metabolic rate is slow and sluggish, the fuel is not burnt quickly so it's stored in the system for a longer period of time. It then gets transported to the excess stores if it hasn't been burnt or utilised. This will generally mean that you put on body fat.

There are many factors that will slow down a metabolic rate:

1) Inactivity/sedentary lifestyle.
2) Continuous dieting.
3) Lack of carbohydrates.
4) Irregular or infrequent food intake.
5) Stress.
6) Depression.
7) Cold environment.
8) Prolonged high intensity exercise.
9) Over exercising.
10) Thyroid conditions.

Think of it as your ultimate nemesis or the 'intelligent twin'. It seems to know everything you do, guess when you are dieting, adapt to everything you do and also overreact to any stress.

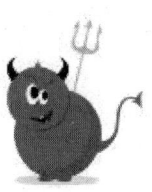

It's almost like having another person lurking in the background trying to see what you are doing! The trick is to take the stress out of dieting and not to let your slow metabolism know what you are doing to it.

If you stress your body, cut its energy, starve it or shock it then it may well guess what you are doing and slow down to protect you.

A slow metabolic rate is one of the most frequent contributors of increased body fat.

Keys to Speeding up the Metabolic Rate

We have covered these briefly before – but just so you have them in a list in front of you, here you are!

These keys are pretty universal for most people and are the basis of the entire structure of the diets and lifestyle which will aid you in reducing your weight – and controlling it.

1) Eat 5–6 small meals throughout the day.
2) Do not cut out carbohydrates for more than 4 days.
3) *Low* intensity cardiovascular exercise, e.g. walking, stationary bike exercise, stepper, cross trainer.
4) Cycled high and low carbohydrate days.
5) Cycled fats in the diet which will vary the amounts of natural fats in the foods you are eating.
6) Change the diet regime every four weeks by following the guidelines in this manual and learning to recognise when you body

is changing its rate.
7) HAVE A CHEAT DAY ONCE A WEEK! REBEL!!!
8) Keep warm – if you are cold the metabolism slows down to conserve energy instead of burning it.
9) Change lifestyle or deal with stress issues.
10) **THIS IS REALLY IMPORTANT:** Deal with depression or negative situations which cause the system to slow. Situations which cause you to be in a negative state, like stress or depression, have a negative effect on the body.

Have you noticed how your breathing rate changes when you get angry and you get a different physical feeling?

Have you noticed how, when a major depression hits, you feel tired and lethargic?

Have you noticed, when you get really enthusiastic about something, your energy levels seem to go right up and it feels like you could do almost anything?

Most people have experienced these feelings and so you know there is a connection between how you feel and how the body responds.

The same goes for your metabolic rate. Due to a chain reaction of chemical releases and signals depending on the situation, your body will react in a particular way.

Stress in particular, in the long term, can continue to produce chemical releases which keep the body in a state of readiness for a major upheaval. So, if you are in a continual state of stress over an extended period of time, then you can imagine how toxic and harmful this can be to you.

Changing situations in your life can seem impossible
Sometimes you can't actually change what is happening BUT you can take action with regards to how you deal with it.

Asking someone to change everything is impractical and even more stressful! This is why the Rebel Day is so important. Not only does it kick the metabolic rate up – it also helps you to start doing something for 'you'.

The philosophy of the Rebel Day is about regaining control, taking one day in the week and making all or part of it yours. It also creates a thought process outside of the other situations you are currently in and creates something which feels more in your control.

Not only does it FORCE you to rebel with your diet, it also forces you to make that time special.

Having dieted all week, the Rebel Day becomes very important and a lot of effort is put into it, effort you do not normally put into something which is for YOU.

You may find that this begins a chain reaction into other areas of your life.

> *'You can't separate peace from freedom because
> no one can be at peace unless he has his freedom'*
> Malcolm X (1925-1965), *Malcolm X Speaks*, 1965

Chapter 10

Nutrition

This is the technical bit about what it is that you are putting into your body.

We are going to cover slow carbohydrates, fast carbohydrates and fibrous carbohydrates, plus your protein and the very building blocks of your body, which are amino acids.

'Why would I even consider reading this section?' you may ask.

Simply, because if you are going to incorporate this diet into your life and be able to manage it on your own, it would be handy if you understood what carbohydrates, proteins and all the variations of them were!

This is very simplified and, if you were a nutrition boffin, you would be tutting at me right now. However, for the purpose of what you want to do, it is easier to split this down into various groups. But, before we do that, let's just try and understand what carbohydrates and proteins actually are.

Carbohydrates

Carbohydrates are components of food that provide a source of energy for the body. We are going to split them into three groups.

Simple or Fast carbohydrates: These are found in fruits and are easily digested by the body. They are also often found in processed foods and anything with refined sugar added. They are also called 'fast sugars'. These include most fruits, cane sugar, maltodextrin powders, sweets etc.

Complex carbohydrates: We are going to split these into two groups for ease of use.

Slow carbohydrates and **fibrous carbohydrates** (or also known in my courses as 'furry carbs'): Slow carbs are found in nearly all plant-based foods, and usually take longer for the body to digest and, therefore, are a wonderful slow-release facility for a sustained, drip feed, effect of energy through the day. They are most commonly found in bread, pasta, rice, potatoes etc.

'Slow carbs' are used more frequently as they tend to fill out meals and are also seen as an essential part of most meals, which in some cases is true.

They are far more effective for slowly releasing fuel into the system and giving you a feeling of having more energy. The ideal way of using them is to provide a small amount per meal, but not enough to completely cover your fuel expenditure, thus forcing your body to start using the fat reserves. You MUST do it in such a way that your body and brain doesn't notice it is happening so you have to 'sneak it around the back door' without the brain noticing and throwing a fit by slowing down your metabolism.

My main gripe is about pasta. For some unearthly, misguided reason, pasta is seen as a healthy choice and 'good for you' in the weight loss industry.

Official Rant

Unless you happen to be a dab hand at making your own pasta or if you buy pure, fresh pasta, your so-called healthy choice has copious amounts of other ingredients, including huge amounts of carbohydrates. It seems to be added to every diet. Why on earth would you do that? As far as I am concerned, pasta is THE SPAWN OF THE DEVIL unless you use very small amounts of it, in which case caution should be applied and it shouldn't be approached unless with a big pointy stick and a full bomb disposal protective suit.

Carbohydrates, in general, provide the cells in the body with the energy they need. When carbohydrates are consumed, the body turns them into glucose, which provides sufficient energy for everyday tasks and physical activity. If the body produces too much glucose, it will be stored in the liver and muscle cells as glycogen, to be used when the body needs an extra burst of energy. Any leftover glycogen that isn't stored in the liver and muscle cells is turned into fat.

If a person is exercising for just a short period of time, say thirty minutes of walking or jogging, the body will release glycogen to be used for energy. If you're exercising for an extended period of time, or doing more strenuous exercise, the body will turn to its fat reserve for energy.

Carbohydrates (complex slow)

1) Porridge Oats
2) Low fat bagel
3) Rice
4) Potatoes
5) Yams
6) Rice noodles
7) Whole meal bread
8) Cereals
9) Egg noodles

10) Pasta
11) Pulses

Fibrous Carbohydrates (furry Carbs)
First of all, the 'furry' carbs business came about from teaching a weight management course and somehow not being able to say 'fibrous' for the entire day. I had to resort to 'furry', which has stuck and, in fact, has found its way into the manual I use for teaching therapists how to deal with weight clients.

Furry carbs are all green vegetables, including green salads and leafy vegetables.

Now, in this type of diet, furry carbs are used for rather a different reason. They have the same properties as Slow Carbohydrates but they also contain fibre, which is largely due to the structure of the plant.

This is harder for the body to break and doesn't provide such an effective and straightforward a carbohydrate supply. However, it does still provide a level of slow carbs, as well and having a higher nutrient level and fibre level.

As this is more difficult to break up, your body has to start working harder to metabolise it. In fact, you burn more energy in breaking it down than what the food actually contains. So, including a furry carb in your meals not only gives you a certain level of slow carbohydrate, but it also gets your body working harder and assists in raising your metabolic rate.

However, if you only lived on protein and green veg you would eventually find yourself getting pretty damn tired, so we still add in small amounts of slow carbs to make sure you have the energy to think and carry out your everyday activities as well as losing weight.

Proteins
A myth about protein is that if you just eat protein, or a diet very high in protein, you will lose weight. This is not the case.

As with anything, if you eat more than you are burning off, unfortunately you will still put on weight. Probably not as quickly as if you just ate flapjacks all day, but you will still put on weight.

The truth about protein-only diets is that you can't stay on them. If you continually only have protein, your body will recognise that you are not giving it enough energy and will begin to slow down. This is why you should always limit the length of time you have any zero carb days, as your metabolism will become slower. Once again, if you overdo it with the amount of protein going in, you will store body fat.

Also, pure protein and lack of carbohydrate has been shown to reduce mental function, resulting in short term memory loss, lack of concentration and mood swings to name but a few. So, be careful.

Proteins are made of strings of amino acids that form chains known as peptides. Our bodies need dietary protein to accomplish many basic functions, such as building bones, moving muscles, and repairing various types of tissues throughout our body. Dietary protein, an essential nutrient, comes from meat, dairy foods, and certain grains and beans.

Proteins differ by the types and order of amino acids they contain. Even though there are only 20 amino acids, they create almost endless variations in chains as long as 500 links.

Proteins form inside animals (including humans) and plants through processes that synthesize peptides. Humans cannot synthesize certain 'essential proteins' and so we must ingest them through food. These essential proteins are made of phenylalanine, threonine, methionine, tryptophan, leucine, isoleucine, lysine, and valine amino acids.

As building blocks for our tissue and a catalyst in metabolism, the jobs of dietary proteins are almost too many to enumerate. Our digestive system breaks down protein to its amino acid constituents. They're involved in the nervous system, repairing and maintaining tissue such as bones and skin, and bringing energy to cells. Dietary requirements vary from 1.4-2.5 oz (40-70 g) of protein per day. Too much protein might deplete calcium, whilst too little causes a form of malnutrition called *kwashiorkor*. Insufficient protein weakens the heart and other muscles, eventually leading to death. Incidentally, proteins are responsible for most food allergies.

Proteins can be found in the following foods:

1) Chicken
2) Eggs
3) Turkey
4) Fish
5) Lean pork
6) Lean red meat (only for use on higher carb days)
7) Tofu
8) Beans

Amino acids
Amino acids are the building blocks of proteins. They band together in chains to form the stuff from which your life is born.

It's a two-step process, as follows.

Amino acids get together and form peptides or polypeptides. It is from these groupings that proteins are made. And there's not just one kind of amino acid.

A total of 20 different kinds of amino acids form proteins. The kinds of amino acids determine the shape of the proteins formed. Commonly recognised amino acids include glutamine, glycine, phenylalanine, tryptophan and valine. Three of those — phenylalanine, tryptophan, and valine — are essential amino acids for humans; the others are isoleucine, leucine, lysine, methionine, and threonine. The essential amino acids cannot be synthesized by the body; instead, they must be ingested through food.

One of the best-known essential amino acids is tryptophan, which performs several critical functions for people. Tryptophan helps induce normal sleep; it helps reduce anxiety, depression, and artery spasm risk; it also helps produce a stronger immune system. Tryptophan is perhaps most well-known for its role in producing serotonin.

Amino acids make up 75 per cent of the human body. They are essential to nearly every bodily function. Every chemical reaction that takes place in your body depends on amino acids and the proteins that they build. The essential amino acids must be ingested every day. Failure to get enough of even one of the ten essential amino acids can result in protein degradation. The human body simply does not store amino acids for later use, as it does with fats and starches. You can find amino acids in many places. In fact, more than 300 have been found in the natural world, from such diverse sources as microorganisms and meteorites.

> *'Complaining is good for you as long as you're not complaining to the person you're complaining about'*
> Lynn Johnston (1947-), *For Better or For Worse*, (2003)

Chapter 11

What rebels are not told

Now then, before we start into the diet design, there are a few things you need to know.

Water, water, everywhere!
Initially, with any diet, because you are cutting out the products that make you hold excess water, such as some types of carbohydrate, salt and a few of the preservatives, you will lose a lot of water. This has a lot to do with processed foods as they are loaded with it.

Many diet plans will claim that this is 'instant fat loss'. Sorry, but physically it can't be. You will, however, start to rapidly lose excess water in the first two weeks, although this does not mean you will be dehydrated. You will just be holding a lower natural level of water because of your diet quality.

Yes, this does mean that you will be making frequent trips to the loo, so please do make a note of service stations and handy hedges on any long car journeys!

Some people can lose up to 7 or 8kgs in the first two weeks if their diet consisted previously of processed foods – so don't be surprised if this happens and, no, it isn't a miracle. After that it will seem to slow down and this will be the body fat starting to come off, so you will be looking at maybe 1kg per week.

Water retention also occurs when you get stressed, are pre-menstruation, or when you eat processed, highly spiced or salty foods. MSG (monosodium glutamate) commonly found in Chinese food is three times the strength of salt and will cause you huge amounts of water retention.

When you have your Rebel day, as a lot of the foods you may eat will be highly flavoured, they may have a lot of water retentive properties. So, do NOT worry if you find you have put on weight after your Rebel day – it's just water and will come off during the week.

Also, if your weight fluctuates suddenly – don't assume its fat. It can't be! It is probably water and with sticking to the diet you can drop this water off quite easily, so don't stress about it.

Oh, and speaking of stress… Stress causes water retention as well, so that's another good reason to deal with your stress levels.

Just to give you an example. These days, when I need to drop weight before a competition (yes, usually I do) to get into my weight category, I will cut out all carbohydrates for 48 to 72 hours. Simply by doing that I can lose up to 3kgs in body weight. The problem is that I lose strength at the same time. However, I weigh in 24 hours before the competition day so, as soon as I weigh in, I pack in carbohydrates, fats, sugars continuously and rehydrate and generally I will be heavier than I was before, because of the deliberate water retention I have aimed to cause.

Cravings – and what to do about them
This is bound to happen at some point and here is what to do.

Most commonly there are sugar cravings. If they are persistent over a period of a couple of weeks and you are very thirsty then I would pop into your GP to have your sugar levels checked.

If they are occasional then you are just having a withdrawal thing happening or maybe you just really fancy a bit of chocolate!

Well – there are a couple of ways of dealing with this.

I'm not going to say eat a piece of fruit, although this is the ideal and perfect way of dealing with it. Sometimes that is just not enough to satisfy the craving.

What I suggest is one of these three things:

1) Eat a piece of fruit or drink some fruit juice (I know – I have to say it!)
2) Have a diet drink. Yes, this has additives and flavourings which are not good for us, but if it helps then do it. It's real life here – not a nunnery.
3) If you do this, your body *thinks* it has had something sweet and sugary, even though it hasn't, so it quashes the cravings.
4) A hot chocolate low calorie drink! Again not ideal but it really does work wonders. Not only does your body think it has had sugary stuff, but your brain thinks it has had CHOCOLATE! Wooohooo! Unfortunately, many of them have a high sodium level so you may have a bit of water retention the next day.

Natural cravings do settle down. When we have had a life of lovely highly flavoured foods and sweet temptations, it's only natural that you will miss those things that give you perceived 'pleasure'.

I do promise you that over a little time, the cravings will settle down and remember – you only have six days before being able to raid the cake shop!

I'm breastfeeding. Can I still use this diet?
At present there isn't any research to suggest that anything contained in this diet would affect your baby through breastfeeding. However, as you will know, as long as the mother has a balanced healthy diet there is no reason for any deficiency to be passed onto the child.

But, if you have any concerns about this, or your own diet, you should always seek a consultation with your medical practitioner or midwife before starting any diet regime.

Although it is sometimes recommended that you intake a higher calorie or higher carbohydrate diet whilst breastfeeding, if you do continue this then it is likely you may put on weight.

Moods
You know, I would love to tell you that there are no mood swings and you will remain on a completely even keel. However, some people do get mood swings. Personally, I don't, as I am so pleased at losing body fat and feel a lot better for it.

However, you might find as your body adjusts that you might get a little bit irritable. This is mainly due to the shift in hormones and chemical changes going on. With the zero and low carbohydrate days you may get a few mood swings but, in reality, because of the length of time you are on it (maximum of two days) it is unlikely that you will. You may feel a little tired and hence a bit grumpy, but that will be it.

Obviously if you are having noticeable mood swings then it may be advisable to adjust your carbohydrate intake a little at a time to see if it is that which is making you 'dragonesque'!

I can't see how I am changing
If you happen to be like so many other people with some low self esteem and confidence issues, it is sometimes hard to see any changes in yourself when you look in the mirror. You know that your clothes are feeling looser, you feel more comfortable, but in the mirror you can't see any difference.

Sometimes, depending on your state of mind at the time, it seems as if you can see a change in how you look by the hour. As we both know, this isn't really possible. So, if this is the case, then put it down to a mood fluctuation, change your self-talk to a more positive language and then have a look. Remember, focus on the positive and how you want to look and be aware of the hard work and effort you are putting into it. Remember to be proud of what you are achieving and the fact you are changing your life.

Frequently, this is just a self-confidence and body perception problem that many people have. You will find that you feel better about yourself as you change small things in your life to reduce stress and take back control and time for you.

To be able to see what you really look like, it really is a matter of taking the very first image you see as you leap in front of the mirror. The longer you stand there, the more the image will distort.

I can remember coaching someone who had awful self esteem at the start. She had been bullied at work quite badly. In fact, with a number of contributing factors, she had suffered a complete breakdown not long before I started working with her.

She was completely amazing. Everything she did was with heart and soul and the transformation was amazing. However, her body was changing faster than her self-esteem and, even though the results were obvious, she just couldn't see it.

She told me about the time she had spent looking in the mirror trying to see the changes which had happened, even though she knew she had come down two dress sizes.

So, I suggested that she sneak up on the mirror, leap in front of it, catch the initial good glimpse and then walk away before her mind had time to start changing the image according to how she felt about herself at the time.

That lady then phoned me to tell me that she had actually seen what she looked like for the first time in years and was nearly in tears – and, yes, it was from being happy, not terror! Using that method she carried on until she could stand and look in the mirror at herself and really feel better about herself, plus get a better view of what she really looked like.

It may sound daft but if this problem rings any bells for you, just give it a try! It's about being one step ahead of your own mind sometimes.

I'm dieting and dropping in size but my weight isn't changing
Well, then that's great.

What can happen over a period of time, especially if you have been eating very few meals, is that you can lose body fat but not lose weight. Too much importance is in fact put on actual body weight. It's about losing the body fat and size, isn't it?

What can happen after the initial 'water shed' is that, because of the balanced diet you are having, all the nutrients and proteins are being used effectively. The protein, especially if you haven't been eating a lot of it, is transported to the tissues that desperately need it. So, for instance, if the muscle tissues have been starved of proteins, the increase in protein will be brawn into the tissues – mostly muscle tissues – and they will become more 'dense'.

This doesn't mean you are putting on muscle, it's just that the density of the tissue is increased. Therefore, as you lose body fat and size, sometimes the density increases which will weigh a little heavier, so your weight may remain relatively static whilst still reducing that stubborn body fat. So – throw away those scales!

> *'What some call health, if purchased by perpetual anxiety about diet, isn't much better than tedious disease'*
> George Dennison Prentice

Chapter 12

The diets & when to use them

This is actually the easy bit!
As I explained before, your diet is going to be five meals a day. There are five different Rebel Diet formats: this section is going to tell you what each of them are, when to use them and WHY!

1) The NORMAL Rebel Diet
This is for normal progressive body fat loss. It gives the body just enough carbohydrate for it to think nothing nasty is going to happen to it and let it carry on working. It initially will allow some excess water to come off and then seem like it is slowing down. That is when the body fat is actually coming off.

It gives you enough protein to feed the body with all the essential nutrients and is also low fat.

So, you will use some of the stored body fat. It is a slow, progressive diet which is easily implemented and you can cheat a bit if you get stuck. Remember, this isn't a restrictive regime.

It can seem a bit bland to start with, especially if you are used to a high salt, processed food type of diet. You could use things like sweet Thai chili sauce, a bit of ketchup, a little bit of low fat mayo etc., just to give the food a bit of extra taste.

I can promise you that the initial blandness for some people will disappear. When your taste buds lose the addiction to the artificial high flavouring, then you start to really taste the natural flavour of the foods you are eating. It can take a week or two, but it will happen. Just use a little extra 'zing' from a condiment to give you that spicy flavour if you need it.

Now, this NORMAL Rebel Diet day is for use in the first four weeks of your diet. Then you go on to cycle the days listed below to keep that old nemesis of the 'slow metabolic rate' from raising its ugly head!

When you have all that done, it's simply a matter of using it when you need to and taking all of this into your own lifestyle and making it work for you. Notice which combination works best for you, feel better about yourself, use the Rebel Day to give momentum to your future and continually giving confidence to your abilities as each week you do something special. It's all a journey of discovery, for your body, mind and future, and it is up to you to make it work.

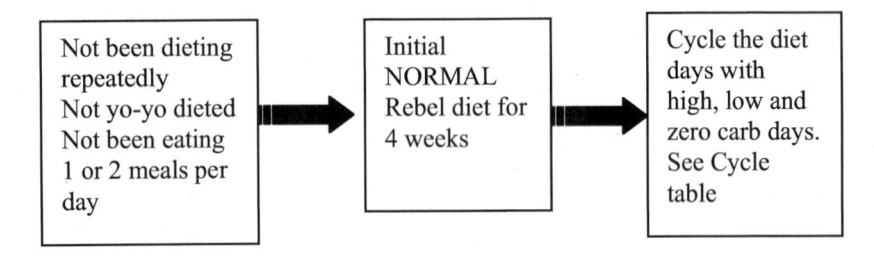

Not been dieting repeatedly Not yo-yo dieted Not been eating 1 or 2 meals per day	→	Initial NORMAL Rebel diet for 4 weeks	→	Cycle the diet days with high, low and zero carb days. See Cycle table

2) *The High Carb Rebel Diet Day (or for two weeks at the start if you have already been dieting)*

There are two ways of using this.

    a)   You can start your diet using this for two weeks if you have been a serial dieter for a long time OR if you have only been eating one or two meals a day for a prolonged period of time and really need to FORCE your metabolism up. This high carb structure is simply to allow your body to return to a normal and faster rate instead of a slow preservation mode; OR

    b)   As a single high carb day when you cycle your diet. Many people find that they lose body fat doing this for a couple of weeks while the body comes out of 'starvation mode' and feels safe enough to return to a higher normal rate. It lulls it into a false sense of security and lets it get all comfy while you wait until you are ready for further subterfuge by implementing another diet style!

The other way of using it is when you have done the initial NORMAL diet for a month and your metabolic rate is slowing down because it has worked out what you are doing.

This is done by cycling days of low and high carbs to completely confuse your metabolic rate - it doesn't know what is going on at all and therefore doesn't slow down.

It's like dealing with a friend who is a bit of a prima donna. If you let them think everything is completely fine while you quietly make changes in the background, keeping everything on an even keel, then you are less likely to provoke a hysterical fit where they lock themselves in a room and won't come out and 'shut down'!

HIGH CARB DIET FOR EITHER:

| First 2 weeks of diet before starting the NORMAL Rebel diet – for those who have been continuously dieting on and off | As one of the cycled days you will be using AFTER the initial NORMAL Rebel diet. This is listed in the cycle table below |

3) The Low Carb Diet Day (part of the cycled diet days)
This is only used when you get to the cycling stage of the dieting. It is never used consistently or else your body will work out what is going on. Low carbohydrate diets work well over a short term, but over a long term they really do mess your system up and it can be very difficult to encourage it to come out of hiding and go back to a normal rate.

Those who have experienced yo-yo dieting or constantly restricted carbohydrates as part of their diet will probably recognise this 'low carb day', as part of the structure of this is not worrying too much about the fat intake.

Increasing the fats for the occasional day is fine, as some of those natural fats are required for healthy body function. It's when you get into the artificial fats and loaded fats from processed foods that you run into trouble.

Using a low carbohydrate day means that you will, on that day, be expending more energy than you are taking in. You will burn additional fat reserves on this day. However, if you continue to use this over three or four weeks, the usual thing happens - you will eventually lower your normal metabolic rate and gradually reduce your effective results.

When you combine this with a series of high, normal, zero carb and Rebel days, then you keep the confusion going; it will reduce overall the energy consumed to energy expended ratio, keep the metabolic rate raised and continually lose body fat.

Remember, that when you finish the initial paper diet, you will have been noticing what you respond to and also altering amounts slightly, depending on what works for you. You will be taking this over yourself and using the combination of days in varying ways and having fun with it.

When I say 'having fun with it' I mean having fun watching what your body does, what weight you lose, when you lose water and when you don't;

seeing what happens when you get stressed or low and really getting to grips with taking over the management of your weight. You'll know when and how to use the diet and having that all important Rebel day to do the things you always wanted to do and really make them happen.

4) Zero Carb Days
Again – this is only used when you are cycling your diet.

I have to warn you that all the people who have done this diet unfortunately seem to look forward to their Zero carb days! This is most disappointing, seeing as this is supposed to be the hardest day AND you should feel pretty tired.

However, the thought of being able to have fried eggs and bacon seems to override any feeling of tiredness and propel you into a state of glee! Bah humbug to you if this is the case for you!

You will only use it down the line of cycling your normal, high and low days. It's the last cycle where you mix zero and high carb days before going back to the start position of the 'normal' diet days for a month.

Once you get through that period then you take the diet on yourself and you use this in combination with the other diet days. It is a highly effective day as, once again, you are taking in less recognisable energy than expending it. The fats, as with the low carb day, are not important in this instance but obviously if you continued with this then the amount of fat consumed would not be good for you at all.

If you use this day where you really are just taking in protein and some fats, then slipping it in for a maximum of two days running, then this can be very effective. However, do watch the fats.

Quite often, by the time you get to this stage of the fixed initial diet, your body fat is down to a maintainable level, or certainly heading that way, and it's just a matter of throwing in some diet days and cycles when and if you want them. We would call this a 'maintenance' diet.

Again – these are NOT to be used consistently as they will mess up all your hard work.

Why would you not use them continually? Prolonged carbohydrate restriction will give you:

a) Slower metabolic rate
b) Reduced ability to think
c) Reduced ability to concentrate
d) Tiredness
e) Irritability
f) Mood swings

g) In severe prolonged restriction your short-term memory can suffer
h) Constipation
i) Susceptibility to illness from lack of natural nutrients affecting your immune system.
j) Lethargy and lack of motivation

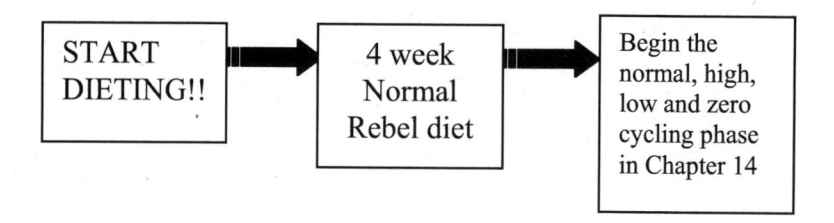

START DIETING!! → 4 week Normal Rebel diet → Begin the normal, high, low and zero cycling phase in Chapter 14

5) YOUR REBEL DAY!

No holds barred unadulterated cake shop day! Why? Well, after six days of any type of dieting, your body – especially if it has a naturally slow metabolic rate – will probably realise something funny is going on and will start to slow down a bit. Also, because you are beginning to use your body's fat reserves as fuel, it will also realise that there may be a situation occurring! This certainly can be the case if you have a sensitive system and have repeatedly dieted in the past.

So, to convince your body that everything in the garden is rosy and to FORCE it to speed up, you are going to take in foods which will be really hard to break down and ask it to speed up to be able to process them. You need to put your calorie counting brain to one side now and work on the principle of speeding up your metabolic rate!

In having to suddenly work really hard to break down all this strange stuff, which will probably include processed foods and naughty nibbles, it has to shift up the gears a number of notches.

In doing this, the metabolism will be raised for a period of time so that, when you start back on the diet the next day with reduced energy intake, the metabolism is still raised and burns at that continued higher rate whilst eating into your fat reserves even more. Most people are a little tentative at first about letting themselves go, so if this the case, then just have a cheat meal in the evening to start with.

Frequently, people who have used the diet express delight that, in fact, they feel they have lost more after their Rebel day than towards the end of the week!

I MUST point out, however, that continued daily use of the Rebel Day will not keep your metabolism high and you will not be thin! It only works when you are using a diet strategy!

> *'A goal without a plan is just a wish'*
> Antoine De Saint-Exupery (1900-1944)

Chapter 13

So, give me the bad news. What *can* I eat?

So – here is the food list
    The list is made up of the options you have, so you can mix and match them as you want. Keep the amounts the same when following the diet until you get to know what works for you and you can take it over yourself.
    Remember, this isn't for ever. This is just to get you down to the body shape you want and then you maintain and adapt it how you want. You won't need to diet all the time, maybe just have one or two days a week low carb and eat relatively clean the rest of the time, but still have the 'naughties' when you feel like it.
    The diets are broken down into SMALL, MEDIUM and LARGE people! As I am not there with you I have to work on a basis of height and make the assumption that the frame of the person is commensurate with height.
    For instance, the intake of food for someone under 5ft 3in should be less than that for someone 6ft 2in. However, if the person under 5ft 3in is very active and the person who is 6ft 2in is very sedentary, then that is where your own common sense must prevail. The diet will still work for both examples; however, it will need to be fine tuned by you throughout its course.
    In the diet sheets you will see an amount in grams for protein, slow carbs and furry carbs. Underneath the diet I will also give you an idea of how much the amount looks like.
    You don't need to weigh out everything to the gram, although initially you probably will need some scales until you will be able to measure how much something is just by looking at it.
    This may seem a bit of a hassle at the start, but it really does become easy and second nature. In some other weight loss programmes they give you meals you can buy or products you can eat, but this means that you are not able to eat what you want and make your own decisions without having to buy a pre made meal.
    With the foods listed below, the emphasis is on 'clean' food, by which I mean food which is not processed and in its original form. That way you know exactly what is in it and can gauge how you react to which diet and

can take it over yourself and adapt it to suit you.

There may be some foods you like which I have not listed here. This does not mean that you can't have them - I may have forgotten to list them, but remember there will be an on-line forum to answer any questions you have. This is about learning how to take this on yourself and incorporating it into your life rather than having me or anyone else telling you what to do!

The sections listed are:

- Protein
- Slow Carb
- Furry Carb

Also, for some of the meals I have added in fruit, but again it is up to you what you have. Initially, for a decrease in body fat the diet regime should be the same. Alterations dependant on results <u>can be done after the four-week initial period</u>.

The design consists of:

- Normal days
- High and low carbohydrate days cycled
- Zero carb days
- The REBEL DAY

<u>PROTEIN</u>

Suggested protein Groups:

- Chicken (any part of the chicken, it doesn't matter. If you want to be fastidious then don't have the skin, but in the grand scheme of things it really doesn't matter that much)
- Turkey (same applies as per chicken. Be careful that you are not buying a processed product, as a lot of turkey products can look like they are raw but are in fact processed and highly salted and flavoured)
- Fish (see below). Buy fresh fish when you can
- Lean pork (straight forward?)
- Lean red meat (only for use on higher carb and zero carb days due to the fat content)

- Tofu (used in its pure form)
- Beans (used as a protein source like a mixed bean salad. Be careful if buying tinned beans as they will have a lot added)
- Quorn (if you must)
- Eggs (you can use egg whites on their own in omelettes or scrambled eggs for pure protein, or the whole egg, although it is higher in fats)

Fish and tinned fish

Just one other point. What can happen is that I will write 'fish' in a diet for someone and then get bombarded with questions about what type of fish. Any type of fresh fish is fine, although it is expensive.

Tinned fish is ok, just watch out for it in brine or oil. The brine is full of salt, which will give you some water retention, while the oil will destroy what you are trying to do! You could have the fish in oil on a zero carb day, but it really is loaded with artificial fats and so it's best to stay away from it. If you are going to buy, for example, tinned tuna, you can buy it in plain water these days which is perfect.

For Vegetarians

Any of the meat products listed in the diets you can substitute with the following:

- Tofu
- Textured vegetable protein (TVP)
- Egg Whites
- Soya beans/lentils/kidney beans/black beans
- Tempeh
- Seitan
- Concentrated soya

CARBOHYDRATES – SLOW

- Porridge Oats (you can make this with water in the microwave or milk in the saucepan; it's up to you if you use full fat, skimmed or semi skimmed)
- Low fat bagel
- Weetabix
- Shredded wheat
- Bran flakes

- Banana
- Rice (any type you like. If you want to be very careful then ideally brown rice)
- Potatoes
- Yams
- Rice noodles
- Egg noodles
- Whole meal bread
- Pasta (if you really have to)

Additions of fruit with two or three of the meals is a good idea to keep cravings at bay.

Obviously this is where common sense prevails. If you are working out what to have for breakfast, there are items in this list which are or are not suitable for breakfast. Conversely, I would not suggest that you choose Weetabix as your carbohydrate source with chicken for an evening meal.

FURRY CARBS

- Any green vegetable
- Any green salad vegetables

As I mentioned before, the furry carbs we have put into a section on their own. The reason for this is that we are using them for a particular job. Not only do they provide you with amazing nutrients, they also give your metabolism a really hard time to break down. So, you tend to burn more energy in breaking down the furrys than is contained in them.

This is one of the reasons why we have them so heavily in the last meal of the day, to keep your metabolism running high through the night when it might normally have slowed a little.

Fibrous Furrys examples (really, it's all the other vegetables so the list is endless):

- Mushrooms
- Tomatoes
- Peas
- Carrots
- Bean sprouts
- Red peppers

- Onions

These are fibrous vegetables which don't necessarily fit in the furry carb section as they have a slightly different content, but you can add these into your pure FURRY quota.

The difference with the fibrous furrys is that they have a different composition to your pure FURRY carbs, so they aren't quite as good at helping to keep your metabolism whirring away.

Protein Shakes

Everyone connects protein shakes with bodybuilders and athletes! However, they have their place in dieting.

Frequently, people will tell me that they feel restricted with when they can eat, either at work or with general timing constraints. It has also been said that while they are getting used to eating so many times a day, they find it hard to eat all of the meals.

One of the options you have is to replace the 'in between' meals with a protein shake. These would be meals 2 and 4 (when you get to the diet structure section).

The reason you would do this is because the better protein shakes just come in a powder form. You buy them in a tub and in various flavours – including CHOCOLATE! You buy a shaker as well and either add milk or water to the powder and it shakes up into a thick drink which does really feel like a small meal.

It also means that you can take it with you in the car, at work, walking or doing anything else where you find that you can't physically eat a meal. It also means you can still have a 'meal' without missing any of the essential components.

Obviously, if you are on a high carb day, you will be losing some of the carbohydrates. So, you can either add a teaspoon of glucose or maltodextrine to the protein powder to add in some carbs OR add some more carbohydrate to one of the other meals of the day.

I would not advise using this as a replacement for any of the meals 1, 3 or 5. However, if you find you are doing this more and more, I would look at your days structure or possibly ask yourself if you would prefer having a drink than a meal? If the answer to that is yes, then you should look at the possibility that you might have the start of an issue with food. This certainly is a rare occurrence, although something which should be asked, nonetheless.

When I recommend protein shakes, of course the first things I am asked are:

1) Where do I buy them?

2) What do I buy?
3) I just looked for a protein powder and there are thousands! What am I supposed to be looking for in a good protein supplement?

First of all, you can either nip into a gym and they will have a store of them. You also have the option of looking on-line at some of the supplement and health food stores. They normally have a discounted range of protein supplements. Many of them will look like bodybuilding supplements, but this is NOT what you are using them for, and NO they will not put muscle on you unless you are training appropriately and really hard to create that look.

When choosing a protein supplement, you are looking for a basic, no frills, does what it says on the tub product. There are a few of these around, like Prolabs's range of Pure Whey which is low cost and good quality. You also have SK Sports range of Vyomax proteins as well.

What you are looking for is something which has NOTHING else added to it. So many of them now have added carbohydrate, added creatine, added vitamins etc.

You are looking for a product which is a pure protein source. Anything which says 'gain' on it generally means there are other supplements in there and should therefore be avoided.

Just a couple of notes about protein powders – some of them also have a high sodium content. This means you may carry a little bit of excess water with them, or possibly quite a lot.

The lowest sodium content product I am aware of is the Vyomax Protein power which, in its unflavoured powder form, contains no sodium at all. However, as a rule of thumb, any protein powder supplement which has close to, or above, 2mg of sodium per 100g protein may give you some water retention.

I remember coming up towards a competition once and as usual I was fighting to get my weight down and keep it down (before I knew better). I had run out of my usual protein and bought a different one (I am not saying which one it was!) and then noticed suddenly that my weight had gone up overnight by 3lbs! I hadn't been aware up until that point that the sodium levels in protein supplements could vary so much; and what surprised me even more was that all my other associates hadn't realised either!

Obviously, if this happens then it isn't body fat, it has to be water. So I looked at the sodium content of this very expensive protein power and found the sodium content was five times the amount of my old one. So, no wonder I had water retention!

So, what do I do now?
Ok, so you are starting your diet today. You have not really dieted continuously for a period of time and haven't been eating one meal a day for the last year? **Then go straight to diet 1.**

If you think that your metabolic rate has slowed down a lot due to stress, dieting or prolonged lack of eating, then you will need to follow the **high carb diet** for 2 weeks.

> *'The only thing that saves us from the bureaucracy is inefficiency. An efficient bureaucracy is the greatest threat to liberty'*
> Eugene McCarthy (1916-2005), *Time* magazine (Feb. 1979)

Chapter 14

The nitty gritty!

In this chapter I am going to list the diets depending on your height. I have to use this as I don't know you personally and therefore I can't prescribe the exact amounts for you.

This book is about being able to take your own diet into your own hands and not needing me or anyone else. The foods listed are a guideline and I don't give you serving suggestions or how to cook them. It's just common sense and a wee bit of thought about what you can do with the foods in the list that give you the ultimate freedom to take charge of your own weight.

Remember – we also have a forum available to you for support and advice, but the whole emphasis is on being able to take control of this yourself and not needing me or anyone else.

However, based on your height we have a rough idea of the amounts to consume but, as I have stated before, you will need to adjust the amounts when you take this over yourself later on. You will lose body fat regardless and will need to notice throughout the diets how you respond to certain combinations. For instance, if you would like to slightly reduce the amount of slow carbs to see if that increases the body fat loss, then try it, but make sure you are not starving your system and reversing all the hard work you have already put in.

Also, remember that if you are 5ft 2in and rushing about all over the place, the amount of energy you will burn up is going to be different to someone who is 6ft tall and who has a very sedentary lifestyle.

It's time to take back the control and get to know YOU.

Break away from the diet companies that tell you what to eat and when. You are unique and it's only *you* that can work out what works best for you.

So, let's begin. Let's Rebel!

REBEL 1 – the starting diet to get you on your way

The First Four Weeks
This is what we call the 'normal' Rebel Diet. This is the mid range, middle of the road one, which you usually start your diet routine with. You can use

this as a base diet and make your alterations later on.

> Page 107: 5ft 3 and under
> Page 108: 5ft 4 to 5ft 8
> Page 109: 5ft 9 and over

REBEL 2 – high carb diet

This is for use during the cycling OR if you have been knicker-dieting and your metabolism has slowed down.

> Page 110 & 111: 5ft 3 and under
> Page 112 & 113: 5ft 4 to 5ft 8
> Page 114 & 115: 5ft 8 and over

REBEL 3 – low carb day

This is only for use during the cycling period. You can throw in a couple of days of this a week which will help you to maintain or lose weight, whenever you want or need to later on.

> Page 116 &117: 5ft 3 and under
> Page 118 & 119: 5ft 4 to 5ft 8
> Page 120 & 121: 5ft 9 and over

REBEL 4 – zero carb day

Same as the low carb guidelines. This is only for use during the cycling period and you can throw in a couple of days of this a week, which will help you to maintain or lose weight whenever you want or need to later on.

> Page 122: 5ft 3 and under
> Page 123 & 124: 5ft 4 to 5ft 8
> Page 125 & 126: 5ft 9 and over

<u>If you are hungry at any point you can drink fruit juice, cordial with added water, diet sodas (although not advisable) and this should help.</u>

<u>If you are stuck and can't get a meal – eat anything, just find the most sensible option</u>

Rebel Diet: Freeing You from Diet Hell

REBEL 1 – under 5ft 3
The normal Rebel Diet
For 4 weeks
only if you have NOT been dieting
OR eating 2 meals or less per day

For the start of your diet and for four weeks. Use this for six days and then your REBEL day on the seventh. This is for normal progressive body fat loss. It gives the body just enough carbohydrate for it to think nothing nasty is going to happen to it and allows it to carry on working.

MEAL 1 (breakfast)
40g carbohydrate
e.g. porridge oats - microwave with water and add honey to taste OR 1 weetabix with skimmed milk and a maximum of 2 teaspoons of honey.

MEAL 2
50g protein
e.g. chicken/turkey/fish
100g furry carbs
Small (size of a side plate) green salad
AND
1 piece of acidic fruit (orange, nectarine, apple etc)

MEAL 3 (lunch)
50g Protein
e.g. chicken/turkey/fish
60g slow carbs (this is dry weight)
e.g. half jacket potato or rice/pasta

MEAL 4
1 piece of fruit – any fruit you like

MEAL 5
100g protein, eg. chicken/turkey or fish
50g slow carb
e.g. half jacket potato (about the size of your fist)
150g furry carbs (pre cooked weight)
e.g. green veg (this is pre-cooked weight and made up of any green veg you like AS LONG AS IT'S GREEN!)

REBEL 1 – 5ft 4 to 5ft 8
The normal Rebel Diet
For 4 weeks
only if you have NOT been dieting
OR eating 2 meals or less per day

For the start of your diet and for four weeks. Use this for six days and then your REBEL day on the seventh. This is for normal progressive body fat loss. It gives the body just enough carbohydrate for it to think nothing nasty is going to happen to it and allows it to carry on working.

MEAL 1 (breakfast)
60g carbohydrate
e.g. porridge oats - microwave with water and add honey to taste OR 1 weetabix with skimmed milk and a maximum of 2 teaspoons of honey.

MEAL 2
70g protein
e.g. chicken/turkey/fish
100g furry carbs
Small (size of a side plate) green salad
AND
1 piece of acidic fruit (orange, nectarine, apple, etc.)

MEAL 3 (lunch)
80g Protein
e.g. chicken/turkey/fish
80g slow carbs (this is dry weight)
eg. small jacket potato or rice/pasta

MEAL 4
1 piece of fruit – any fruit you like

MEAL 5
120g protein
e.g. chicken/turkey or fish
60g slow carb
e.g. small jacket potato (just smaller than the size of your fist)
150g furry carbs (pre cooked weight)
e.g. green veg (this is pre-cooked weight made up of any green veg you like AS LONG AS ITS GREEN!)

Rebel Diet: Freeing You from Diet Hell

REBEL 1 – 5ft 9 and over
The normal Rebel Diet
For 4 weeks
only if you have NOT been dieting
OR eating 2 meals or less per day

For the start of your diet and for four weeks. Use this for six days and then your REBEL day on the seventh. This is for normal progressive body fat loss. It gives the body just enough carbohydrate for it to think nothing nasty is going to happen to it and allows it to carry on working.

MEAL 1 (breakfast)
80g carbohydrate
e.g. porridge oats - microwave with water and add honey to taste OR 1 weetabix with skimmed milk and a maximum of 2 teaspoons of honey.

MEAL 2
80g protein
e.g. chicken/turkey/fish
100g furry carbs
Small (size of a side plate) green salad
AND
1 piece of acidic fruit (orange, nectarine, apple etc)

MEAL 3 (lunch)
100g Protein
e.g. chicken/turkey/fish
80g slow carbs (this is dry weight)
e.g. jacket potato or rice/pasta

MEAL 4
1 piece of fruit – any fruit you like

MEAL 5
140g protein
e.g. chicken/turkey or fish
60g slow carb
e.g. half jacket potato (about the size of your fist)
200g furry carbs (pre cooked weight)
eg. green veg (this is pre-cooked weight made up of any green veg you like
AS LONG AS IT'S GREEN!)

REBEL 2 – 5ft 3 and under
The High Carb Day
Part of the Cycle Pg 128
OR for 2 weeks prior to Rebel 1 if you have been dieting already
OR eat 2 or less meals per day

There are two ways of using this.

You can either actually start your diet using this for two weeks if you have been a serial dieter for a long time and really need to FORCE your metabolism up.

OR: Incorporate it into your high, normal, low and zero mixed combination.

If you do use this at the start of the Rebel Diet, you can still use it when you are combining the different carb days so you can have the best of both worlds!

MEAL 1
60g slow carbohydrate

e.g. porridge oats - microwave with water and add honey to taste
OR 1 weetabix with skimmed milk and a maximum of 2 teaspoons of honey with a banana OR
2 slices whole meal toast & 1 piece fruit OR
60g of muesli with full fat milk
OR any other cereal of your choice 60g

MEAL 2
50g protein & 60g slow carbs

e.g. Chicken salad sandwich – using whole meal bread (no butter)
OR small rice salad with mixed beans – 60g beans and 60g rice
AND 1 piece of fruit NOT banana

MEAL 3
60g protein

eg. beef, pork, chicken – don't worry about the fat content on this day
80g slow carbs
e.g. pasta, yam, rice, wholemeal bread

If vegetarian, choose your higher fat meat equivalent and use 100g.

MEAL 4
2 pieces of fruit – banana if you like

MEAL 5
80g protein
e.g. beef, pork, chicken, bacon, lamb either grilled, ground in a burger or any other way you want
80g slow carbs (pre cooked weight)
e.g. rice noodles, egg noodles, pasta etc., half baked potato etc.
150g furry carbs
the green veg thing

REBEL 2 – 5ft 4 to 5ft 8
The High Carb Day
Part of the Cycle Pg 128
OR for 2 weeks prior to Rebel 1 if you have been dieting already
OR eat 2 or less meals per day

There are two ways of using this.

You can either actually start your diet using this for two weeks if you have been a serial dieter for a long time and really need to FORCE your metabolism up.

OR: Incorporate it into your high, normal, low and zero mixed combination.

If you do use this at the start of the Rebel Diet, you can still use it when you are combining the different carb days so you can have the best of both worlds!

MEAL 1
80g slow carbohydrate
e.g. porridge oats - microwave with water and add honey to taste
OR 1 and a half weetabix with skimmed milk and a maximum of 2 teaspoons of honey with a banana
OR 2 and a half slices whole meal toast & 1 piece fruit
OR 80g of muesli with full fat milk
OR any other cereal of your choice 80g

MEAL 2
50g protein & 80g slow carbs
e.g. Chicken salad sandwich – using wholemeal bread (no butter)
OR small rice salad with mixed beans – 50g beans and 80g rice
AND 1 piece of fruit NOT banana

MEAL 3
60g protein
e.g. beef, pork, chicken – don't worry about the fat content on this day
100g slow carbs
e.g. pasta, yam, rice, wholemeal bread

If vegetarian, choose your higher fat meat equivalent and use 100g.

MEAL 4
2 pieces of fruit – banana if you like

MEAL 5
80g protein
e.g. beef, pork, chicken, bacon, lamb either grilled, ground in a burger or any other way you want.
80g slow carbs (pre cooked weight)
e.g. rice noodles, egg noodles, pasta etc., half baked potato etc.
180g furry carbs
the green veg thing

Emma James

REBEL 2 – 5ft 9 and over
The High Carb Day
Part of the Cycle Pg 128
OR for 2 weeks prior to Rebel 1 if you have been dieting already
OR eat 2 or less meals per day

There are two ways of using this.

You can either actually start your diet using this for two weeks if you have been a serial dieter for a long time and really need to FORCE your metabolism up.

OR: Incorporate it into your high, normal, low and zero mixed combination.

If you do use this at the start of the Rebel Diet, you can still use it when you are combining the different carb days so you can have the best of both worlds!

MEAL 1
100g slow carbohydrate
e.g. porridge oats - microwave with water and add honey to taste
OR 1 weetabix with skimmed milk and a maximum of 2 teaspoons of honey with a banana
OR 3 slices whole meal toast & 1 piece fruit
OR 120g of muesli with full fat milk
OR any other cereal of your choice 80g

MEAL 2
60g protein & 100g slow carbs
e.g. Chicken salad sandwich – using wholemeal bread (no butter)
OR small rice salad with mixed beans – 60g beans and 100g rice
AND 1 piece of fruit NOT banana

MEAL 3
80g protein
e.g. beef, pork, chicken – don't worry about the fat content on this day
120g slow carbs
e.g. pasta, yam, rice, wholemeal bread
If vegetarian, choose your higher fat meat equivalent and use 100g.

MEAL 4
2 pieces of fruit – banana if you like

MEAL 5
100g protein
e.g. beef, pork, chicken, bacon, lamb either grilled, ground in a burger or any other way you want.
120g slow carbs (pre cooked weight)
e.g. rice noodles, egg noodles, pasta etc., half baked potato etc.
220g furry carbs
the green veg thing

REBEL 3 – 5ft 3 and under
The Low Carb Day
Part of the Cycle Pg 128

This is only used when you get to the cycling stage of the dieting. It is NEVER used continuously.

MEAL 1 (breakfast)
60g protein
e.g. 4 egg whites (cooked any way you want) or 60g bacon OR 2 egg whites and 30g bacon
20g slow carbs
e.g. half slice wholemeal toast OR 20g (dry weight) of porridge oats with water and honey to taste

MEAL 2
60g protein
e.g. chicken/turkey/fish
60g furry carbs
e.g. small (half size of a side plate) green salad
AND
1 piece of acidic fruit (orange, nectarine, apple etc.)

MEAL 3
80g protein
e.g. chicken, pork, tuna
100g furry carbs
e.g. small green salad (size of small side plate) OR 100g green vegetable – use a little light dressing if you want to
AND
30g nuts – anything you like NOT SALTED!

MEAL 4
1 piece of fruit – NOT BANANA!

MEAL 5
Protein: 100g
e.g. chicken, pork fillet, salmon etc.
150g furry carbs
Dry weight green vegetables and add some seasoning or light sauce/spice to it. Add in some fibrous carbs as well if you want

to add something to the taste
AND
1 piece of acidic fruit e.g. Orange, apple, pear etc

Emma James

REBEL 3 – 5ft 4 to 5ft 8
The Low Carb Day
Part of the Cycle Pg 128

This is only used when you get to the cycling stage of the dieting. It is NEVER used continuously.

MEAL 1 (breakfast)
80g protein
e.g. 5 egg whites (cooked any way you want)
OR 40g bacon and 3 egg whites in an omelette
40g slow carbs
e.g. 1 and a half slice wholemeal toast with honey
OR 40g (dry weight) of porridge oats with water and honey to taste

MEAL 2
60g protein
e.g. chicken/turkey/fish
80g furry carbs
e.g. small (3/4 size of a side plate) green salad
AND
1 piece of acidic fruit (orange, nectarine, apple etc.)

MEAL 3
100g protein
e.g. chicken, pork, tuna
120g furry carbs
e.g. small green salad (size of small side plate) OR 120g green vegetable – use a little light dressing if you want to
AND
50g nuts – anything you like NOT SALTED!

MEAL 4
1 piece of fruit – NOT BANANA!

MEAL 5
Protein: 120g
e.g. chicken, pork fillet, salmon etc.
200g furry carbs
Dry weight green vegetables and add some seasoning or light sauce/spice to it. Add in some fibrous carbs as well if you want to add

something to the taste.
AND
1 piece of acidic fruit e.g. Orange, apple, pear etc.

'Those who know how to win are much more numerous than those who know how to make proper use of their victories'
Polybius (205 BC-118 BC)

Emma James

REBEL 3 – 5ft 9 and over
The Low Carb Day
Part of the Cycle Pg 128

This is only used when you get to the cycling stage of the dieting. It is NEVER used continuously.

MEAL 1 (breakfast)
80g protein
e.g. 5 egg whites (cooked any way you want) or 40g bacon and 3 egg whites in an omelette
60g slow carbs
e.g. 2 slices wholemeal toast with honey OR 60g (dry weight) of porridge oats with water and honey to taste

MEAL 2
60g protein
e.g. chicken/turkey/fish
100g furry carbs
e.g. small (size of a side plate) green salad
AND
1 piece of acidic fruit (orange, nectarine, apple etc.)

MEAL 3
100g protein
e.g. chicken, pork, tuna
140g furry carbs
e.g. small green salad (size of small side plate) OR 140g green vegetable – use a little light dressing if you want to
AND
50g nuts – anything you like NOT SALTED!

MEAL 4
1 piece of fruit – NOT BANANA!

MEAL 5
Protein: 140g
e.g. chicken, pork fillet, salmon etc
250g furry carbs
Dry weight green vegetables and add some seasoning or
light sauce/spice to it. Add in some fibrous carbs as well if you want to add

something to the taste
AND
1 piece of acidic fruit e.g. Orange, apple, pear etc.

REBEL 4 – 5ft 3 and under
Zero Carb Day
Part of the Cycle Pg 128

Again – this is only used when you are cycling your diet. You will only use it far down the line of cycling your normal, high and low days. Also, on these days, don't worry about the fat content!

I have added some fruit and furry carbs in there, as zero carb days can give you constipation. Keep it in or take it out, however strict you want to be. I know the addition doesn't quite make it 100 per cent zero carb, but it's not that far off it and we want to keep you healthy and sane.

MEAL 1
60g protein
e.g. 4 egg whites cooked however you want.
OR 60g of red meat (this can be bacon, sausage – anything you like)

MEAL 2
60g protein
e.g. 60g of red meat ideally but use chicken/turkey/fish or a meat substitute for the vegetarians. You could have some cheese or something similar with that if you want and add a little ketchup or sauce.
AND
1 piece of fruit

MEAL 3
80g protein
e.g. 80g of chicken/turkey or fish or a mixed bean salad with some light dressing or maybe 40g of each.

MEAL 4
1 piece of acidic fruit
50g nuts (if you have a nut allergy then substitute with either mixed beans or a small green mixed leaf salad about the size of a side plate)

MEAL 5
120g protein
This can be made of anything you want and cooked any way you wish. Have fun! Use a condiment if you want to
100g furry carbs
green vegetables – take your pick and use your imagination!

REBEL 4 – 5ft 4 to 5ft 8
Zero Carb Day
Part of the Cycle Pg 128

Again – this is only used when you are cycling your diet. You will only use it far down the line of cycling your normal, high and low days. Also – on these days, don't worry about the fat content! By the way, I have added some fruit and furry carbs in there, as zero carb days can give you constipation. Keep it in or take it out, however strict you want to be. I know the addition doesn't quite make it 100 per cent zero carb, but it's not that far off it and we want to keep you healthy and sane.

MEAL 1
80g protein
e.g. 6 egg whites cooked however you want.
OR 60g of red meat (this can be bacon, sausage – anything you like)

MEAL 2
80g protein
e.g. 80g of red meat ideally but use chicken/turkey/fish or a meat substitute for the vegetarians. You could have some cheese or something similar with that if you want and add a little ketchup or sauce.
AND
1 piece of fruit

MEAL 3
100g protein
e.g. 100g of chicken/turkey or fish or a mixed bean salad with some light dressing or maybe 40g of each

MEAL 4
1 piece of acidic fruit
60g nuts (if you have a nut allergy then substitute with either mixed beans or a small green mixed leaf salad about the size of a side plate)

MEAL 5
140g protein
This can be made of anything you want and cooked any way you wish. Have fun! Use a condiment if you want to
120g furry carbs
green vegetables – take your pick and use your imagination!
You may also feel tired on this day – this is quite normal as you are taking away your energy reserve.

REBEL 4 – 5ft 9 and over
Zero Carb Day
Part of the Cycle Pg 128

Again – this is only used when you are cycling your diet. You will only use it far down the line of cycling your normal, high and low days. Also – on these days, don't worry about the fat content! By the way, I have added some fruit and furry carbs in there, as zero carb days can give you constipation. Keep it in or take it out, however strict you want to be. I know the addition doesn't quite make it 100 per cent zero carb, but it's not that far off it and we want to keep you healthy and sane.

MEAL 1
100g protein
e.g. 6 egg whites cooked however you want
OR 60g of red meat (this can be bacon, sausage – anything you like)

MEAL 2
80g protein
e.g. 80g of red meat ideally but use chicken/turkey/fish or a meat substitute for the vegetarians. You could have some cheese or something similar with that if you want and add a little ketchup or sauce
AND
2 piece of fruit

MEAL 3
120g protein
e.g. 120g of chicken/turkey or fish or a mixed bean salad with some light dressing or maybe 40g of each

MEAL 4
2 pieces of acidic fruit
60g nuts (if you have a nut allergy then substitute with either mixed beans or a small green mixed leaf salad about the size of a side plate)

MEAL 5
160g protein
This can be made of anything you want and cooked any way you wish. Have fun! Use a condiment if you want to
180g furry carbs
green vegetables – take your pick and use your imagination!
You may also feel tired on this day, this is quite normal as you are taking away your energy reserve.

Chapter 15

Confuse that Nemesis!

After the initial four-week diet, you are now moving into territory where your body might be working out what you are doing. The lowering of body fat may be ringing alarm bells and there is always the risk at this point that your metabolic rate may start to slow down.

What we do to keep everything raised is to start to cycle low and high carbohydrate days for two weeks and then cycle high, low and zero days for a further two weeks after that. Of course, you have the legendary Rebel Day every seven days to keep you SANE!

As stated below, the cycle is to keep your body confused as to what you are doing, a stealth attack, and you need to keep that going once you have done the basic Rebel 1 diet.

Once you have done the twelve weeks, then you are equipped to deal with the cycling yourself and play around with it to see what suits you best.

You can also put in normal days as well or just drop a couple of low or zero carb days into a week of just normal eating to maintain or decrease body fat. That's all it takes you know – it's not complicated. Getting to know what suits you best is the bit that takes a little time.

You will notice at the end of each week a change in your body and then you can keep a note of which combination gave you the best results. Then, when you cycle everything on your own, you can stick to that combination for a while, do three days a week dieting and the rest eating what you want. Play around with the amounts and just have fun with it whilst building up confidence in how you look, having your Rebel Day and changing your life.

Cycling Your Diets
OK. Here is the cycle for someone who isn't doing the high carb speed-up at the start of the diet:

First 4 weeks: NORMAL DIET – Rebel Diet 1

Remember to have your Rebel cheat day on the seventh day of each week. Also, your cheat day does not have to be on a Sunday – this is only an example. Just as long as it is the seventh day in the cycle.

Next 4 weeks: HIGH/LOW – Rebel Diet 2 and 3

H = high carb day Page L = low carb day Page

Mon	Tues	Wed	Thur	Fri	Sat	Sun
L	H	H	L	L	L	**REBEL**
H	L	L	H	H	L	**REBEL**
L	L	L	H	H	L	**REBEL**
H	H	L	H	L	L	**REBEL**

Following 4 weeks: HIGH/LOW/ZERO

H = high carb day L = low carb day Z = zero carb day

Mon	Tues	Wed	Thur	Fri	Sat	Sun
H	Z	L	H	L	Z	**REBEL**
Z	L	L	H	Z	L	**REBEL**
H	Z	H	L	Z	L	**REBEL**
Z	L	H	L	H	Z	**REBEL**

So – now you have the structure. This is for twelve weeks. Once you have done this then you will have noticed the difference on how your body responds on different days and different cycles.

Once you finish the diet cycle of twelve weeks
THEN TAKE A WEEK OFF!!!

When I say a week off, I mean eat whatever you want, whenever you want and do not worry about anything. Why? Because no matter how you dress it up, you have been dieting for twelve weeks. Mentally you will be tired and need a break and you deserve it.

How do I cycle after this diet?
Well, that is very much up to you, but here are a few guidelines that will help you:

- Never do more than three low carb or zero carb days in a row
- Always make sure you have a Rebel Day if you are doing a full week's diet
- Remember, it isn't a prison, so if you really want something then

have it
- DO go out to dinner, there will always be something you can have and even if there isn't exactly what you should have, what the hell?!
- Remember to have a break of at least a week if you diet for twelve weeks consecutively
- Watch how you react to certain combinations and keep or dump them
- If you are not doing six days a week diet and just dropping in a few diet days, don't use the Rebel Day
- If you notice a certain combination of days gives you some water retention and you aren't comfortable with it – change it

Some examples of cycling periods after you have done the Twelve week Rebel Diet would be:

N= normal non-diet days
H= high carb days
L= low carb days
Z= zero carb days

Mon	Tue	Wed	Thur	Fri	Sat	Sun
N	H	Z	Z	L	L	**REBEL**
Z	L	H	N	N	L	N
L	L	H	H	Z	L	**REBEL**
N	Z	L	Z	N	N	N

If You Have Had A Break
If you got down to the weight you wanted and have had a break for a period of time, maybe put a little weight on or feel that you would like to continue to change your shape, then make sure your metabolism hasn't slowed down at that point.

You will know, from getting acquainted with your body, whether or not your system has slowed or if you have returned to any old habits, like not eating enough through the day. So, all you need to do is go back to the four-week diet structure of the normal diet and you will probably have worked out any changes to amounts you need to make.

Follow that for the four weeks and then go into the cycling mode again. You may not have to do the high and low days on their own, just go straight into the normal, high, low and zero mix. Just as an example, you could (see next page):

```
                    ┌──────────────┐
                    │ Had break    │
                    │ from diet    │
                    │ and would    │
                    │ like to do   │
                    │ more         │
                    └──────────────┘
                           ↕
┌──────────────┐                    ┌──────────────┐
│ Begin        │                    │ Start the 4  │
│ cycling      │                    │ week         │
│ again with   │  ←──────→          │ normal       │
│ normal,      │                    │ Rebel diet   │
│ zero, high   │                    │ just to get  │
│ and low      │                    │ everything   │
│ days         │                    │ moving       │
└──────────────┘                    │ again        │
                                    └──────────────┘
                           ↓
                 ┌──────────────────────────┐
                 │ Return to maintenance    │
                 │ structure and enjoy life │
                 │ and naughtiness          │
                 └──────────────────────────┘
```

Have you reached the weight or body fat level you want?
If you have reached your desired body shape? Then this is what you do now.

To maintain body fat levels, what we suggest is that you keep your diet as 'clean' as possible. This means trying to stay away from processed foods and junk foods.

Try to keep the meals small through the week and still have your

CHEAT REBEL DAY one day a week.

You can also incorporate three days a week on the 'normal diet' from our Rebel Diet and then three days just eating clean, PLUS have your Rebel Day on the seventh day. This will generally keep everything at a sustainable level and you should be able to maintain what you have lost.

Remember, you can still go out for dinner, have the odd chocolate bar if you want it, have a life and live your life and sustain the body fat level you want.

I would strongly suggest still keeping up some kind of cardio vascular exercise. You can, if you want, drop the frequency down a bit to three days a week, but I would hope by now that you would miss it if you didn't do it!

Also, it really is a good idea to keep this up for your own health and the 'feel good' factor it gives you. It is also a bit of 'you' time as well, where nothing can touch you, and that time is completely yours.

> *'That is what learning is. You suddenly understand something you've understood all your life, but in a new way'*
>
> Doris Lessing

Chapter 16

Exercise

Here we go again with the metabolic rate shut down thing.

Think of it like this. As with the dieting, you don't want to rock the boat and give your body a tip-off that you are trying to lose body fat. So, it's the same approach with the training or exercise.

I'm mainly only going to discuss cardio vascular work at the moment, as this is the main key to the body fat loss. Also, most of you aren't going to be an obsessive gym rat like me! For the purpose of the book, I only cover cardio vascular exercises, as going into any other training would not only over-complicate everything but possibly overload you completely when, in fact, it is very simple.

Obviously, if you do want to go to the gym then please take care. If you wait a little, then I should have something out which will help you train. In the meantime, just start off gently and build up so everything feels achievable and you gain confidence from being able to do each step.

If you do 'high intensity' cardio vascular work, for example, anything that will raise your heart rate above 60% of its resting rate will risk causing shut down to your metabolic rate. Of course, this is not always the case and you could add some high intensity work in here if you wish, but it really isn't necessary at this stage.

This is where I am going against a lot of material out there, but from experience and working with many clients with a stubborn metabolism I have found this more effective.

For people with a 'normal' metabolism that isn't slow or 'over sensitive', then short burst high intensity or cycled high intensity work can be great for body fat loss

If you have an over-sensitive system, when you blast your body and put it under stress, it will slow down to conserve energy and lower your metabolic rate. Again, it can work short term, but over a period of time it will contribute to slowing the metabolic rate.

So, although it means you have to do lower intensity exercises for longer, it will sneak the work in without your system realising what you are doing and allow you to lose the body fat. Yes, it is slower to a degree, but better than causing 'shut down' and ruining all the hard work you are putting in.

Doing the CV work (cardiovascular work) in the morning *before* eating raises the metabolic rate through the day and then at night, before you go to bed, it keeps it ticking over at a higher rate while you sleep. However, be sure not to do it just before you go to bed or else you won't be able to sleep!

The various types of low intensity CV work I would suggest are:

- Stationary bike (great for at home)
- Walking (treadmill or outside and can be done at home without having to go to a gym)
- Stepper (you can buy small home steppers)
- Vacuuming the home!
- Tai Chi or other slower and more intense classes or home workout

Of course you may well have other suggestions which I haven't thought about, so test it out.

A few of these suggestions are things you might have to get up a little earlier for in order to do them, or you might not be able to do them until after breakfast if you have a hectic family life. Don't worry, if you want to do it then you will make sure it happens. There is always a way, although you may have to put your foot down with others to ensure you have the peace and time to do it. Sometimes, in doing this, it begins the process of taking time out for yourself and starting the journey of creating the life that you would like, even if you aren't living in a mansion in Beverly Hills!

From personal experience, while I was learning about how to be flexible with my own body and the fact that it seemed to like doing its own thing, I had been told to do all this high intensity work. Initially it was working, but then it seemed that the more I pushed, the less body fat I would lose. I would take in even less carbohydrate but STILL nothing was happening.

Of course, everyone assumed I must be cheating on my pre-competition diet, as they said I couldn't possibly be doing all that work on so little energy and not lose body fat.

They hadn't considered that my metabolic rate had almost shut down and so my body was furiously hanging on to everything that went in.

This is when my own self-confidence took a major nose dive. The people who were helping me were losing faith in me. But what was more frustrating was that they thought I was lying about sticking to my pre-competition diet and doing the CV work I had been set. It was then that I thought I would 'go quiet' and do things my own way, which I had done years before.

I dropped the high intensity work, did an hour walking at 5am in the morning and 10pm at night with my walkman on, put the carbs back up and 'voila!' - the body fat started to come off again. When I went to competition and won, I didn't tell them I had changed everything they were telling me to do and, of course, they took credit for my success. It seemed easier not to tell them and then just take things into my own hands after that.

Remember, the body fat level I needed to get down to was well below where you are looking to go, so you don't need to do what I was doing, just in case that routine fills you with dread. Also, I was training for two hours a night as well to get down.

So far, with all the people I have worked with, when something hasn't been working as well as it should, rather than assuming the client is lying to me, we always adjust amounts and play around with the amounts of carbs vs protein, plus the CV work and we have always got a result. As long as they were honest with me, that they had maybe had a day where they just wanted pizza and had it or had a few other blips, but it very rarely made a difference. It was a change in the basic diet and CV work that made the difference.

To start with on Weeks 1 & 2
(for 5 days a week, choose your own days): 15 minutes morning and evening.

Weeks 3 & 4
20 minutes morning: Before your first meal
20 minutes evening: After your last meal and not too close to going to bed.

Weeks 5 and 6
(for 5 days per week, choose your own days)
30 minutes in the morning and evening

Week 7
No cardiovascular work at all

Weeks 7, 8 & 9
(for 5 days per week, choose which days but keep them in the order listed below)

Day 1: 30 minutes morning and evening
Day 2: 20 minutes morning and evening
Day 3: 40 minutes morning and evening

Day 4: 10 minutes morning and evening
Day 5: 20 minutes morning and evening

Why am I cycling this?
For the same reasons you will already be cycling the diet, we are starting to cycle the CV exercise. The body starts to become conditioned to what you are doing and will 'normalise' to the work load you are asking it to do. So, we start asking it to do something different so it doesn't begin to second guess what you are doing.

Weeks 11, 12, 13 and 14
(for 5 days per week)

Now, I am asking you to take this over yourself.

- For 5 days do your CV work, vary the times
- Keep the time ranges between 10 minutes and 40 minutes
- Do no more than one day at 10 minutes
- Do not go over 40 minutes per session
- Fit the timings in with the day's schedule you have – this way you are starting to take this over yourself and incorporate it into your own lifestyle and schedule

Once you have gone through this diet and scheduled bit, again you will notice what you have the best results with. If you push yourself too much you are risking your body working out what you are doing and, remember, there is no rush with this.

Take notice of what combination of CV and diet gives you the best results and also notice where the body fat is coming off the most first.

Bottoms
Yes, I know this is a favourite subject for many people. So, I just want to tell you a couple of secrets about bottoms.

First of all, you ladies out there may have noticed that before your period you might get water retention; your waist, lower abdominal region, thighs and bottom seem to expand. This is quite normal and takes a few days to subside.

We girls tend to hold water in this region and so, if you need to drop that water or keep the water down during that time then when you are cycling, keep the carbs down and use the low and zero days.

You may notice when you start dieting that it's the bottom half that seems to reduce quickly. This is normally where the water comes off first and then the body fat will start to reduce after that. So, don't get distraught if you find that suddenly you put on weight in that area, as it's probably water.

If you want to tone that area, or your bottom, then you just have to do your cardiovascular work on a slight gradient. Walking, incorporating a slight gradient, will help firm that area. Slightly increasing the tension on a stationary bike will help also. This is part of what we call 'spot reduction', which has been poo-poohed at by others who don't believe in it. However, from personal, professional and research experience, it damn well does work if done correctly.

One thing you need to realise about your bottom is that it is a huge muscular area. You have a couple of main muscles there that do a lot of work all the time. So, when you exercise them or do a few exercises designed to tone and firm them, they do so under the body fat which is there. In other words, you won't see the real benefit unless you reduce the body fat over them. Just like getting defined abdominals, you won't see the definition until you reduce the covering.

A simple Exercise
Now then, here is a very effective exercise that you can do in your spare time which will make a HUGE difference. It's called ballet kicks. It lifts the buttocks and gives you that curved bottom look instead of the landslide look!

1. All you have to do is face a wall, standing up straight. Make sure your feet are pointing straight and that you are about 4 or 5 inches away from the wall as in fig 1 on next page.
2. Keeping your leg straight – bring it backwards and clench your buttock at the same time. As you bring it backwards, make sure your foot is in a straight line, fig 2 on next page. As you raise it backwards, do it slowly over a slow count of one…two…three…
3. Then hold it when you come to the 'point of tension', fig 3 on next page.
4. This is when you feel the slight burn of the muscle working. Hold that position for another count of one…two…three…
5. Then lower back to the ground, again counting one…two…three…

If you do this at some point during the day, preferably when no one else can see you, then this will start to change the shape of your bottom.

Each day, do it eight times in a row with one leg and then eight times in a row on the other leg. Do that three times. It really is a simple routine.

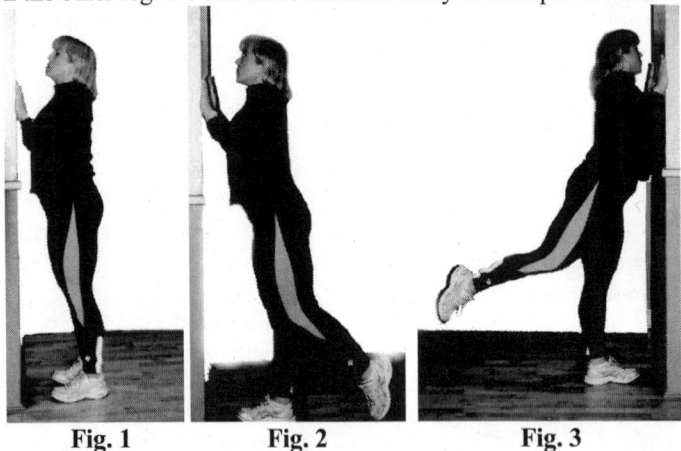

Fig. 1   **Fig. 2**   **Fig. 3**

Bingo and Batwings
I wish I could tell you that this is simply dealt with by reducing water – unfortunately it isn't.

The amount of people I have seen doing the very simple exercise completely wrong makes me shudder with rage! RAGE I tell you!

What is more, they spend time and effort doing it but it is not going to give them any benefit whatsoever. Sad but true.

Some basic points:

1) If you don't feel it working – it isn't working.
2) If you swing the movement or do it fast then you may as well go and have a chocolate éclair.
3) If you don't hold the movement at the point where it is working the most – then you won't feel it work WHICH MEANS it isn't working.
4) Most exercises should be done with a one… two… three… count on the initial movement to the maximum point. Then held for a count of three while tensed and THEN returned to the resting position to the count of three.
5) Little exercises like this will NOT put muscle on you – just tone what you have.
6) Use a mirror when you can, to see what you are doing. It is amazing the angles and strange movements we can produce

without realising it when we can't see what we are doing. (After 25 years of training, I always use a mirror to make sure I am doing the exercise correctly.)
7) Always keep your back straight and bend from the hip rather than with your lower back.
8) Any weight you use, keep it REALLY light. If you are at home doing this, just use a can of beans or a small coffee jar, etc. It's about the *squeeze* and if you are doing it properly you will feel it intensely with virtually any weight. (Most people you see doing this with a lot of weights are swinging it and trying to be flash rather that actually getting results. You find these types in most gyms.)

The Exercise that works
Here is one simple exercise which is commonly called tricep kickbacks. This works the tricep area, which is the bit at the back of the arm that swings about when you don't want it to.

The result of doing this is that it firms and tones the muscle, which means it doesn't swing around as much, even if there is body fat or some loose skin there. So it will improve whatever is there, regardless. Obviously, depending on what is on top of that muscle will determine the final result.

Ok, so here is how you do it:

1) Find an object which is like a bench. Long enough to get your knee and hand on when you bend over and low enough to have your knee on it comfortably.
2) You are going to exercise one arm at a time, so turn side on to the bench with the side you are NOT going to use first.
3) Put your knee on the bench with the other leg straight.
4) Lean forward, keeping your back completely straight and bending from the hip; put your hand flat on the bench (this is the same side as the knee you have on the bench – i.e. if your right knee is on the bench, you will put your right hand down as well).
5) At this point your other leg is straight and your other arm is hanging down straight, fig 1.
6) With the weight in your hand (no vodka bottles please!), fig 2, raise your arm to the start position where your shoulder to elbow is in a straight line; your body and your elbow to wrist is pointing straight towards the floor. The position your arm from shoulder to elbow is in will now NOT MOVE AT ALL throughout the entire exercise. It will not drop, sink, drift outwards, jig up and down or any other

movement which would precipitate a swift rattle to the back of the head with a rolled up newspaper!

7) Now, slowly with a count of one... two... three... raise your hand backwards, fig. 3, until your arm is locked tight and *squeeze* hard and count to three again. You will feel the back of your arm squeeze.
8) Slowly lower your hand back to the start, fig 2, position and pause before beginning the next repetition.
9) Do this for a minimum of eight repetitions.
10) Now, turn around so you do the same for the other side.

This exercise needs to be done in three sets of eight repetitions for each arm.

Repetitions are the number of times you do the movement (otherwise known as 'reps'). A set denotes the number of times you do the group of reps.

If you experience excessive pain or feel any strain outside of reasonable muscle usage for the exercise, stop doing it.

If you have any previous injury or condition which may be aggravated by this exercise, then please consult your doctor prior to commencement of this exercise.

These tricep kickbacks exercises sound complicated when they are written down, when in fact they are very straight forward, so here are some step-by-step pictures.

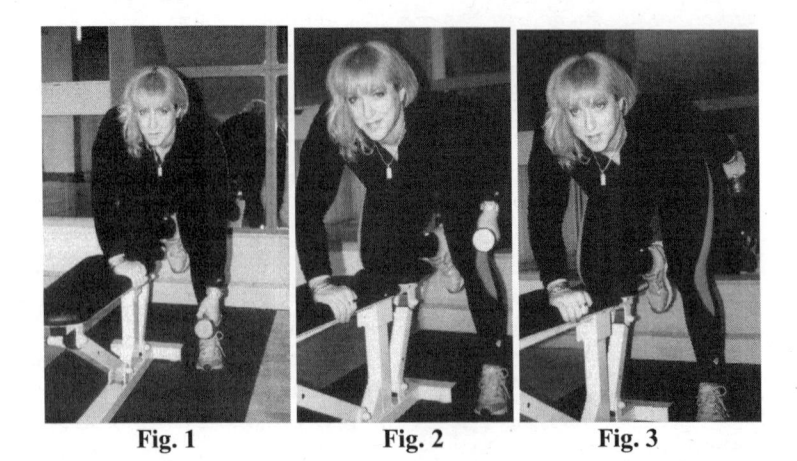

Fig. 1 **Fig. 2** **Fig. 3**

Rebel Diet: Freeing You from Diet Hell

Abdominals

This is one of my favourite subjects.

When I injured my back at the World Championships in 1996, I damaged three discs and had some pretty severe pain which I had to find ways of getting around to be able to rehabilitate myself.

I had been told I would never compete again and probably wouldn't be able to train or carry on in my job. It was like a red rag to a bull at that point; I used my experience and qualifications to rehabilitate myself and go on to win the World Championships in 2000.

However, along the way I had to work out other ways of doing some exercises that were just too painful for me to do in the conventional way.

One of them was doing abdominal work. When I started to experiment, I found a more effective way which had no lower back movement and was producing better results for me and also for my clients. So – this is perfect for you if you have a lower back problem.

Ok, you need to think about your abs as two sections:

Lower abdominal area, which is the old 'pot belly', running from the belly button downwards. The upper area from the diaphragm to your belly button

You know what the key is? Breathing.

When you breathe out, right to the very end of the breath and then try to push more air out, you feel your muscle tighten, don't you? Well, if you do it enough, it may almost feel like cramp. That's what you are looking for with this exercise.

One thing I must advise, **please don't do this** if you suspect or have anything wrong with your neck without checking with your GP first. You know the usual line now: always check with your physician prior to any new exercise.

HELD CRUNCH (No, this is not like any crunch you have done before).

1) Lie flat on the floor. Bend your knees upwards while maintaining contact on the floor with your feet. Don't bring your knees up too much; quite simply, if you don't feel this exercise working, lower your knees an inch at a time until you do, fig 1.
2) Put both hands across your lower abdominals so you can feel them working OR just in front of your face. I usually end up looking like I am praying. Do NOT put them behind your head please.
3) Slowly start to push air out through your mouth and then begin to roll your head towards your chest.
4) As you roll your head towards your chest, your shoulders may

come off the floor slightly - don't let them come right off the floor.
5) Keep pushing the air out really slowly. When you can't move any further, hold that position. Fig 2, and push every last bit of breath out until you feel that clenched feeling almost as though you are about to get cramp.
6) Lower your head slowly back to the ground, fig 1, relax for a moment, breathe in and then repeat.
7) This is a painfully slow exercise but MASSIVELY effective if done correctly – don't rush it.
8) You only need to do eight reps and three sets of this.

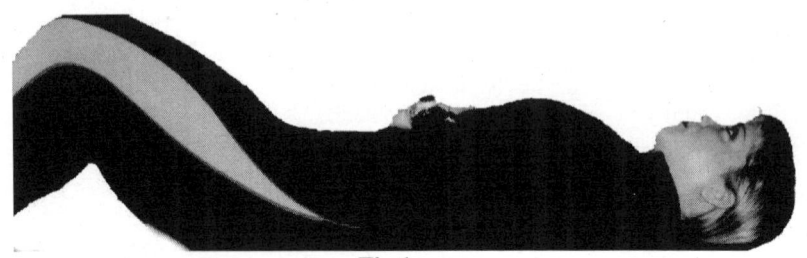

Fig.1

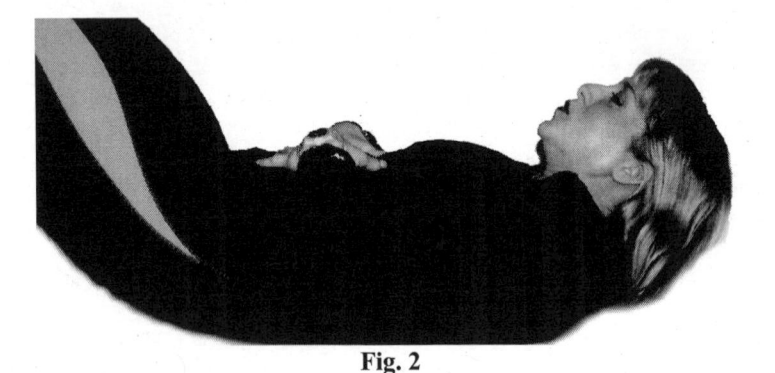

Fig. 2

This is a fraction of all the exercises you could do, but this book is about your life and your diet so I have only covered a couple of common problems and some very simple movements to deal with them.

If you want to go to the gym OR already train at the gym
I could be here all day telling you some do's and don'ts for training at the gym, but for the purpose of this diet I'm going to keep it simple.

One popular misconception is that you will put on a lot of muscle if you go to the gym. This is a total myth. My own physique has come about from 24 years of hard training and 21 years of competing – so unless you want to go down this path, it will never happen.

If you already train, then just carry on with what you are doing. Athletes also use this diet and use it in conjunction with their training. If you already have a routine or are training for something sport specific, then just do what you do.

However, if you are going to the gym to lose body fat and increase fitness, these are a few guidelines:

- Keep the weight light
- Keep the repetition range between and 12 and 15 per set
- Keep the sets to around 4 or 5 per exercise
- Don't leave your rest time in-between sets any longer than a minute

You are looking for a slight burning sensation in the muscle – this means you are starting to tone.

While you are at the gym, if you want to incorporate the CV work, then that is fine. Even if it is after your first meal or before your last – if it works in your schedule, then that's fine. It's all about doing what works for you.

Monsters or kittens?

Unfortunately, gyms are not like they used to be. Years ago, if you went to a gym, you got help from the people who worked there who had probably been training for years and really knew their stuff from practical and personal experience. There was never a personal training environment where people relied on others to get them motivated.

Your training programme was written by the owner or the staff. You never had to pay for individual attention as this was what the gym was all about, plus a sense of community.

Now, the chain gyms ask you to pay for extra individual attention or have kids working there who don't have the incentive or real knowledge to give you the attention you deserve with the payment of your membership.

If you are going to hit a gym, hit the oldest bodybuilding gym you can find. Do not think twice about the others training there, especially if you are a beginner. The people who are real trainers will be helpful, respectful and pleased to see someone who is starting out, training hard and only wants to lose a bit of weight.

One gym I trained at produced top class athletes and many of us were not what you would have called small! It had a hard core gym reputation, but also had a reputation for helping complete beginners regardless of age, build or desired dimensional results.

So, we had women aged 60 plus amongst 20-stone, muscle-bound warriors, with the guys cooing over them and making sure they got the best advice to drop the 10 pounds they set out to lose. Those ladies got advice worth thousands of pounds and were looked after by the best. A word of advice: the bigger the monster they are, the bigger the kitten they are!

I Need To Lose Weight Before I Can Go Into A Gym...
I hear this all the time. Remember, you are going there to do light CV work and some very basic light exercises. You are not going there to build muscle, not to put on weight or size, but just to get out of your environment and into a productive one.

No one will be looking at you. Please bear in mind that each person in that gym is there for their own goal and are not that interested in anyone else. If it is a professional gym with a lot of people who compete there, I can assure you that they are so infatuated with their own training and how they look to really pay much attention to how you look.

Some of the large chain gyms are heaving with people who are not really motivated and also have a little bit of a chip on their shoulder about how they look. You know the type, you meet them every day in life. They seem to spend most of the time looking at and criticising everyone else as it helps their self esteem, yet they don't do anything about their own situation.

This is another reason why I am suggesting, if you do want to go to a gym right now, then look for one a little bit off the beaten track that has some serious people who train there. Those people are dedicated to what they are doing and appreciate seeing someone obviously determined to make changes, as they are doing that themselves and not just making a token gesture. They will appreciate more the effort you are making and are much less likely to make any kind of judgment apart form offering to help.

So, forget the 'I need to lose weight before I go into the gym because everyone will think I am too overweight to be there'. The only person thinking that will be YOU.

People are far too wrapped up in themselves to be worrying about others. BUT, if they *are* looking at you in an unfavorable way, then ask yourself 'What is wrong with that person's life that they need to do that?' OR 'Are they looking at me with respect for being here?'. We can make so many assumptions about what others are thinking and most of the time we are WRONG!

Let me tell you a story.

One day I was heading to the gym and stopped at the petrol station. I was wearing a training vest top and shorts.

There were two women talking by their car as I was filling up my car with petrol and they were looking over. I didn't take a lot of notice.

As you know, I am a bit of a muscly lady so I am used to getting looks and stares. However, as I was standing in the queue to pay, I looked out onto the forecourt and to my horror saw the two women pointing in my direction and squinting at me as they did it.

As my blood was nicely simmering and the hair had gone up on the back of my neck, they walked in to pay for their petrol and joined the queue behind me.

I turned around and said to them 'Do you really need to be so rude? You stood there pointing at me so obviously and do you have any idea how that felt?'

The two women stood there with their mouths open, truly shocked, and said, 'I'm so sorry dear, we were looking at the two for one offer on the doughnuts just behind you.'

Obviously, I then had to continue in the queue with these women behind me wishing that the ground would open and swallow me up, but I hope this gives you an example of how we make huge assumptions of others on a very regular basis.

Do take a personal stereo/MP3 player or something similar with you. It blocks out conversations, keeps you motivated and helps if you are nervous about going in there. Also, if you are going to be doing just CV work, it keeps you uplifted during that time, which can get a bit boring unless you have someone interesting to watch while you are training!

Personally, for CV work I take something with a good beat to it to keep in time with the music. No one notices and, sad but true, I have added extra time onto CV-only workouts because I was enjoying the music so much! Even if you find that hard to take in, try it and you will see what I mean.

A Little Bit Of Advice About Treadmills...
These things can be very varied and sent to try our technical abilities. So, if you get on one, or any other CV equipment for that matter, and it looks like a mystery from ancient Egypt, just hop off and ask someone how to operate it. Most people in the gym will have been through the same thing, so never worry about that.

When you are on a treadmill in a gym, the temptation to look around is amazing. Only look forward and continue looking forward if someone tries to talk to you while you are on there. Ask them to come and stand in your line of sight if they wish to persist in talking to you, as it is so easy for your feet to go in the wrong direction if your head turns and the next thing you know you are being propelled off the back of the machine!

If you are with a friend, then make it clear that you can talk and not look around at the same time if they are on another piece of equipment beside you.

Stick a towel on the rail or somewhere close to you to keep sweat from getting in your eyes. If you can't see, you can't see where your feet are going, which is the fastest way of coming off a treadmill!

If you are in posh gym and there are TVs in front or beside the CV equipment, always choose the equipment which has a direct line of sight to the TV. If you choose anything which is to the side of you or above you, again you run the risk of continually watching the screen with your head turned or tilted…and not your feet!

This advice is designed to save you from the indignity I have experienced from the mistakes I have made, and if you talk to people who have used CV equipment for a long time they will probably tell you stories of daft things that have happened to them as well.

Overall…

Choose what you would like to do. Do a little exercise at home or walking. If you choose to go to a gym to get out of the environment you are in to get motivated, don't feel intimidated - be aware that people are generally more interested in themselves than anyone else Most of all – enjoy it!

> *'There's no easy way out. If there were, I would have bought it.*
> *And believe me, it would be one of my favorite things!'*
> Oprah Winfrey (1954-), *O Magazine*, (February 2005)

Chapter 17

Sympathetic Supplements

Sympathetic Supplements
   This is a difficult subject due to the restrictions on what you are supposed to say and not say and the possibility of me or my publisher getting sued!
   The reason this subject annoys me is because of the amount of conflicting information, governmental interference and regulation, hijacking and misrepresentation from companies wanting to make a fast buck and so-called 'experts' who never allow for the variant of 'individual' response to a basic, naturally-occurring simple vitamin, mineral or supplement. Of course, not forgetting that everything apparently has a paper attached to it saying it gives you cancer. I mean, really..!
   So, for those of us who have reason, the ability to think and use logic along with a large dose of common sense…I will move swiftly on.
   There are few basic supplements which would be considered sympathetic to your body. They generally assist in overall wellbeing, tissue repair, immune system maintenance and upkeep of our bodies to function at an optimal level. Some of these have also been found at some stage to have the additional benefit of lending themselves to helping your body metabolise or burn body fat in some small way.
   Now, nothing is a miracle, none of them are going to give you size zero overnight, although every little bit helps, but they will assist you in improving your overall physical health.
   A word of caution though. Always consult your GP before you take anything, ESPECIALLY if you are already suffering from any condition or taking medication. It is always better to check and, if you are taking anything, if you feel unwell or just 'not right', then stop taking everything. Either consult with your doctor or take one item over a period of time methodically, until you find what it is that is causing the problem.
   Dosages of supplements: you should ask your retailer or qualified advisor for the correct dosage. They should ask you about your current exercise, medical conditions and medication before directing you accordingly. If they don't, take your business elsewhere.

So, below is a short list of some very basic supplements which have the added advantage of 'allegedly' aiding weight loss – and why.

Vitamin C
Vitamin C is a water-soluble vitamin needed for the growth and repair of tissues in all parts of the body. It is necessary to form collagen, an important protein used to make skin, scar tissue, tendons, ligaments, and blood vessels. Vitamin C is essential for the healing of wounds and for the repair and maintenance of cartilage, bones and teeth.

Vitamin C is one of many antioxidants. Vitamin E and beta-carotene are two other well-known antioxidants. Antioxidants are nutrients that block some of the damage caused by free radicals, which are by-products that result when we metabolise what we eat. The build-up of these by-products over time is mainly responsible for the aging process and can contribute to the development of various health conditions such as cancer, heart disease and a host of inflammatory conditions like arthritis. Antioxidants also help reduce the damage to the body caused by toxic chemicals and pollutants such as cigarette smoke. (note to the cigarette smokers out there!)

Vitamin C deficiency can lead to dry and splitting hair; gingivitis (inflammation of the gums) and bleeding gums; rough, dry, scaly skin; decreased wound-healing rate; easy bruising; nosebleeds; weakened enamel of the teeth; painful joints; anemia; lowered immune system efficiency; and, possibly, weight gain because of slowed metabolic rate and energy expenditure.

A severe form of vitamin C deficiency is known as scurvy, which mainly affects older, malnourished adults and you may remember sailors in time gone by had problems with this.

The body does not manufacture vitamin C on its own, nor does it store it. It is therefore important to include plenty of vitamin C-containing foods in one's daily diet. Large amounts of vitamin C are used by the body during any kind of healing process, whether it's from an infection, disease, injury, or surgery. In these cases, extra vitamin C may be needed.

Low levels of vitamin C have been associated with a variety of conditions including hypertension, gallbladder disease, stroke, some cancers, and atherosclerosis (the build-up of plaque in blood vessels that can lead to heart attack and stroke; conditions that are caused by atherosclerotic build-up are often collectively referred to as cardiovascular diseases). Eating adequate amounts of vitamin C in the diet (primarily through lots of fresh fruits and vegetables) may help reduce the risk of developing some of these conditions. There is not much medical evidence, however, that vitamin C supplements can cure any of these diseases.

Obesity and Weight Loss

Studies suggest that obese individuals may have lower vitamin C levels than non-obese individuals. Researchers speculate that insufficient amounts of vitamin C may contribute to weight gain by decreasing metabolic rates and energy expenditures. Many sensible weight loss programmes will be sure to include foods rich in vitamin C, such as plenty of fruits and vegetables.[3]

Chromium Picolinate

Chromium is a terribly difficult area. There have been debates, lawsuits, conflicting research and data about it. As yet I haven't seen one report which has been completely agreed upon by the varying academic research institutions which clearly state, unopposed, that chromium would aid body fat loss, either with or without a controlled diet and exercise regime.

So – how does chromium work?

Chromium picolinate is a nutritional supplement that works to increase the efficiency of insulin to optimum levels. It is a naturally occurring mineral found in minute quantities of foods like meat, poultry, fish, and whole-grain breads. Tiny amounts of chromium are needed to aid the transportation of blood glucose across cell membranes and, if you have a deficiency in chromium, this can lead to damage of insulin-dependent systems. If you have an insulin imbalance, then this finds it hard to regulate the levels of and, therefore, the usage of glucose (energy) in the system.

Again, how chromium picolinate in fact works is speculative and, once again, I think that it has to come down to what you think works for you. You will either try it and believe it is having an effect or not. Personally, for me, I think it has a mild effect and others I know feel the same way, but you are going to have to make your own mind up about this.

One official study claimed that:

> 'After eating, the human body secretes the hormone insulin. In general, the primary function of insulin is to transport glucose to the body's cells in order to provide energy that facilitates cell functioning. It is speculated that chromium picolinate works by stimulating the activity of insulin, thus significantly aiding the body's glucose and fat metabolism, managing the breakdown of glucose and fat.'[4]

---

[3] Further information regarding research into this can be obtained from the Federation of American Societies for Experimental Biology and is based on reports by Sarah Goodwin.

[4] Krzanowski, J.J. (1996). Chromium picolinate. Journal of the Florida Medical Association, 83(1), 29-31.

Kelp
There is a huge amount of controversy about this. Kelp is termed as a 'sea vegetable' and contains high quantities of iodine. Iodine is essential in your thyroid function. Although most people in the UK do not suffer from iodine deficiency, iodine does assist in the regulation on the thyroid gland.

However, some experts say that taking kelp does not assist in weight loss. Some say that it assists in speeding up metabolism. From my own experience, it does seem to have had some effect. However, this is a pretty controversial subject and you should be extremely careful before using this, as it does have an effect on the thyroid function – so please, *please* always see you GP before taking this or any other supplement.

Zinc
Zinc plays an important role in the proper functioning of the immune system in the body. It is required for the enzyme activities necessary for cell division, cell growth and wound healing. It plays a role in the sensory acuity of smell and taste. Zinc is also involved in the metabolism of carbohydrates and can be useful, not only for your own immune system, but also to aid metabolic function and general health.

Vitamin E
Vitamin E is a major anti-oxidant nutrient that inhibits cellular aging due to oxidation (a change in a chemical composition). It supplies oxygen to the blood which is then carried to the heart and other organs. This assists in alleviating fatigue; aids in bringing essential nutrients to cells; prevents the red blood cells from destructive poisons; assists in dissolving blood clots; has also been used by doctors in helping prevent sterility, muscular dystrophy, calcium deposits in blood walls and heart conditions. There is a universally recommended dosage of 200 IU per day - although this goes up and down like nobody's business and I am not supposed to tell you what dosages to take! You are supposed to consult with your GP and get them to tell you according to current government guidelines.

Green Tea Extract
Green tea extract helps with thermo genesis and aids in the metabolism of fat. Known for years as a powerful antioxidant, it may also be helpful in shedding fat. The most obvious benefit to dieters is that it works without increasing the heart rate, which is most often found in diet aids. The increased heart rate leaves dieters jittery and eventually most dieters stop using the supplement and gain weight back. Now, through using green tea extract, dieters get the weight loss benefits without any of the jittery effects,

especially in obese individuals with hypertension and other cardiovascular complications.

Of course, as with almost everything, there are conflicting reports that state that this is just a placebo, it is a psychosomatic effect and if you believe it to work, it will work. Do you know what? If it works for you, regardless of the findings of whether it does or it doesn't, just let the rest of them fight it out and do what works for you.

Carnitine

Carnitine, also known as L-carnitine or levocarnitine, is made from the amino acids lysine and methionine (you may have seen these bandied around the weight loss circuits). Lysine is also marketed separately as a weight loss aid. However, I haven't seen much evidence or spoken to anyone who used it and found it effective.

Personally, I have used Carnitine at times when I have really needed to lose some weight, along with other supplements, and have found its inclusion was useful. However, this may have been due to the level of my training which had meant I was then deficient in it. So, I can't give you any firm reason why it has specifically worked for me.

It usually comes in a liquid form and is quite expensive, in the £25 to £40 region, but obviously depending on volume and branding.

It helps in the consumption and disposal of fat in the body because it is responsible for the transportation and breakdown of fatty acids. It is often sold as a nutritional supplement. It is found in the highest concentrations in red meats like beef, lamb and mutton and usually in good enough quantities to supplement our diets naturally.

According to William R Sukala, MS, CS, from Wellington, New Zealand, who has carried out research on Carnitine, if you are not naturally deficient in Carnitine then it will not have a significant effect. If you are deficient for some reason then you may see a slight difference in body fat reduction and it could be a useful addition to your own diet and exercise.

You will, of course, come across many more supplements and variations on the market. Just remember, that most natural or herbal products will have a number of supporting or derogatory reports which have been done about them and it will pretty much come down to whether you want to try them or not.

If you follow these simple guidelines then you can't go too far wrong:

- If in doubt, don't buy it
- Always check with your doctor first

Another method of attack is your local health food store. If you can find a small, family or privately-owned shop which seems to have been around forever then usually it means that, whoever is running it, has kept afloat by keeping loyal business and have not killed anyone by the advice they have given! They are generally more than happy to help you with any questions or queries, even if you have a question about something you have seen on the internet. Quite often they will have some kind of nutritionist or equivalent qualification.

They will also be able to help you with exact dosages and guidelines, as well as contraindications for using certain types of natural supplementation if you have a pre-existing medical condition and/or are on medication.

Brands
There are a multitude of brands on the market and it can become very confusing indeed when trying to discern which to buy.

The one company I found to be the most reliable and had consistently won awards, was the most helpful on the phone and had a really good reputation amongst my own peers in the competitive field, was Solgar.

If it seems like I am unashamedly singling them out, well, I suppose I am. From the age of 15 years I have taken natural supplements, which I have found benefitted me greatly in my personal and competitive life, as well as my professional cognitive career, and have certainly felt it when something wasn't working as it should, as you become very attuned to how your body is responding at any given time. This was mostly due to the physical stress of the level of training I had to perform, and still do.

This was the only company I knew of which made no apology for the price of their products as they always sought out the best quality raw components and poured money into its own research. You always knew you were getting the best quality possible when you bought from this company and that is still the case today.

Just to give you an example. I had someone who worked for Solgar on one of the NLP courses I was teaching. He was there for his own personal development, so I didn't know who he worked for when he joined the course.

About two days into the course, I found out who he worked for and nearly dropped to my knees. Having stifled my enthusiasm and got through the rest of the day's teaching, I then cornered him.

I told him about the days when we were starting out in our competitive careers and usually working full-time as well, so money was tight. It was well known that the people who were the World Champions and record holders used only the best and Solgar was one of them.

He wasn't aware at all about how revered his company was, so I thought I would share a bit more with him. I went on to explain that usually none of us could afford to buy all Solgar products in those days, so we would pick out what we felt was most beneficial to us. We would buy those from Solgar and then buy the rest from the other cheaper brands which we knew were of a lesser quality.

What really knocked him for six was when I told him that most of us had gone without, not bought certain foods we needed or something we should, just to be able to afford it. Mind you, I did wonder whether he thought I was angling for a trade discount so I quickly made a point of saying how pleased I was he was on my course!

You may well have certain brands of your own that you prefer and stick with and, of course, that is great. It's just something a lot of people ask me about so I thought it was worth mentioning. Unfortunately, it isn't like TV when you mention a brand and you get thousands of items pouring through your letterbox from the company!

As usual, find what works best for you, take appropriate advice and listen to your doctor – not the marketing campaigns!

Chapter 18

Where do I go from here then?

Once you have gone through the diet in its 'regime' format and worked out what is working for you the best, then you can use this diet with its normal, high, low and Rebel days whenever you need to.

What will have happened is you will have become very aware of how your body responds to different sections of the diet, noticed when you have water retention, seen the differences after a Rebel day, seen the different speeds at which you lose body fat at different sections of the diet and may have noticed and felt the differences between your metabolic rate speeding up and slowing down.

You will also have made changes to your life and outlook which will have a direct result on your body and metabolic responses, enabling you to make the mental and physiological changes you need to take the whole area of weight management into your own hands.

When you have watched and understood what is happening, this makes the job of carrying on with life and maintaining the body you want much simpler than relying on others to tell you what to do or having to buy pills and potions continuously.

The fact that you can drop into a diet section when and if you want it, increase or decrease your CV work and work all of this around your own life, with all its ups and downs, gives you freedom and flexibility.

As well as this, you have also been able to get that 'me' time back and start to create and put energy into an area of your life. That can be the beginning of a total chain reaction to regaining some elements of your life.

Help is always at hand if you need it

There will be an online forum at www.myrebeldiet.com which is full of advice, sharing experiences and question and answer sections. This gives you continuing support, if you want it, throughout the whole process. If you need help or just want someone else to talk to, there will always be someone there.

Of course, there is more extensive information available on training, dieting and more explanations and cycles and things for you to try on-line and also in forthcoming material, to take your experience and achievements to the next level if you wish to.

If you would rather not share or 'go public' on-line then you can always email me! Yes, believe it or not an author who actually responds to emails!

However, there really is everything you need right here unless you want to push your weight management or physical look to the next level or increase your exercise, which is where the further books will come in.

The main thing is to watch how your body responds to different sections of the diet and be able to spot when your metabolic rate is starting to drop. When you then use this diet structure yourself and incorporate it into your lifestyle, you will be able to tell when it is slowing down and you will know exactly what to do and when to do it.

You have the tools here to be able to work with and manage anything to do with your weight. However, always remember to get a GP checkup before you start and at regular intervals just to make sure you are at peak health at all times!

You may in fact fancy coming off all diets for a while and go on a splurge! Well, when you want to lose body fat again, you can now do it easily and without stress.

Be well, be happy and BE A REBEL!

'No price is too high to pay for the privilege of owning yourself'
Friedrich Wilhelm Nietzsche

Troubleshooting Rebel

Commonly asked questions:

1) What happens if I am stuck somewhere and can't eat one of my meals?
Then eat anything. It is actually better to eat something, even if it goes against everything we have talked about, than to not eat at all. If you travel a lot, get into the habit of picking up fruit juice or water, nuts, fruit or a flapjack so you don't miss a meal.

2) What happens if I break my diet?
Well, if you break it then you need to ask yourself – for what purpose did I break it? Find out if you are having sugar cravings! Or if it is a self-motivation issue, then identify at what point you don't appear to be worth the effort?

If you break your diet – don't panic, just go back to where you left off and carry on. If you continue to break your diet – then allow yourself something special each day. It means you will slow down your progress, but that is better than never getting there at all. We are all human.

3) What happens if I have to go out for dinner?
Well then go! Most restaurants will be able to accommodate you and you just pick something which is closest to what you should be having. Just ask them for a portion of rice or salad or baked potato OR ask them to keep the sauce off your fish or chicken. You could just choose whatever you like and is roughly what you might be having anyway. It really is easy and don't stress about it.

4) What about if I have continual sugar cravings?
Ok – one of two things are happening. First you need to go to your GP and get checked for any blood sugar issues. If nothing shows up, then do these two things:

1) Add a little carbohydrate into your diet – especially if you are on the mixed zero carb phase.

2) Use either a diet sweet drink or BEST OF ALL a low calorie hot chocolate drink. It fools the body into thinking it has had something sweet when it fact it hasn't actually had the sugar.

5) I work at a place where I find it hard to find the time to go out and have my meals. What do I do?
There are a few things you can do. First of all you could swap the second and fourth meals for protein shakes and drink them at your desk. Protein shakes are great for filling you up and replacing the protein content you need. However, remember you are not getting any carbohydrate with them so do remember to make sure you have your carbs on the meals you are supposed to outside of that.

See Chapter 13 for information on protein supplements, when and how to use them and also for advice on what to look for when buying them.

6) I seem to be losing a lot of weight very quickly
Again, with this, first of all check with your GP and stop the diet. Sometimes during the first couple of weeks, the weight really drops off as this is water coming off. If that is all clear, then carry on with the diet and take a note of when it happened. If you have made some substantial life changes and are really motoring on with projects and goals, your natural adrenalin will increase and burn more energy and increase your metabolic rate. Notice when you are losing the most weight and when it slows down.

Some of the biggest differences are noticed, not so much from parts of the diets, but when psychologically you make changes to your outlook. This helps your metabolism return to a better and more natural rate for you.

If this happens for more than four weeks continually after the initial four week start period, then add a little more carbohydrate into your diet and see what happens until it stabilises. Remember, if in doubt, see your doctor.

7) What happens if I keep losing momentum?
You need to look at all the things that you will have to do or face if you continue on the diet. Will you have to start talking to people, go to more social networking, do more outside the house? Do you see this as a constant line of hard work for you? (Remember, this is not how this diet system works!)

Go back over the first seven chapters and look at all the changes you could make to get to the place you want to be to really take advantage of what your life has to offer. There may be other things you need to consider, like what may change or what you are frightened you would change around you. Until you address these issues then no diet will work for you.

Use your Rebel Days wisely and work through the week planning on what you WILL DO for yourself and what changes you can make on that day in your life. This is about freedom – not prison.

8) Will I recognise the portion sizes eventually?
Yes, you will. You could also buy some smaller plates as well which 'fit' the size of your portions so you get used to knowing by sight how much you need to have. It's a bit of a pain in the bum initially but you will get used to it. Once that happens, everyone will be amazed and you will be cooking like Gordon Ramsay, knowing the exact quantities by vision!

9) I lost weight but looked in the mirror and wondered 'Is this the best I am ever going to get?'
Ah, that old chestnut, the self-esteem and body image issue! Read over the body image chapter and ask yourself if the image that you see is really reality? If you believe it is, then I would wonder what your self-esteem was like if you could not congratulate yourself on your achievement?

Again – put the Rebel Day to good use as this will help focus you on your goals and doing something positive and productive FOR YOU!

Also, remember that sometimes body fat comes off in places we don't realise and we can't really see!

10) I am getting nighttime cravings, what should I eat?
Those nighttime cravings are a killer, aren't they?! The trouble is, the temptation to grab something quick is just too easy, especially if it's cold and you are floating around in nighttime attire!

Grab a piece of fruit, a couple of strips of chicken, a hot chocolate low calorie drink or fruit juice. More than likely you will be having a sugar craving, so just follow the advice about cravings in number 4 earlier on.

11) I am getting cravings when I get upset – what can I do?
This is what we call comfort eating. You can read about it and what to do in Chapter 7. It is also known more commonly as emotional eating, which really dresses it up in a frilly frock and over complicates it.

12) I have been doing some CV work and have found that I am aching a bit. Is there anything I can do?
Initially, your body will need to get used to the change in physiological demand and will have to adapt, so there may be a period of a few aches. Obviously, if it persists you should check with your doctor. However, some supplements can help with this, like Glucosamine, cod liver oil and vitamin

E. Everything should be taken with advice and a good health food shop will always be able to advise you properly. Licensed homeopaths are also a good complementary accompaniment to dieting and can help with this. They will advise you on which supplements could be useful for you specifically.

13) I get bored with the foods, what can I do?
Get bored? A wee bit of Tabasco, a home made tomato salsa, a dollop of Thai chili sauce, a glug of ketchup, balsamic, garlic, onion, salt, low fat vinaigrette, added onions dry fired with no oil, rice boiled up with tomatoes and black olives - the list goes on. It's endless! Use your intelligence, imagination and creativity, which I know you have as you bought this book! Use the guideline and add a little bit of 'you'. Have fun with this.

14) It all looks very complicated!
It's only as complicated as you would like it to be. The really complicated bit is understanding yourself, but those tools have been given to you in the chapters before the actual diet section! The actual diet is really straightforward, it's just the high and low days which are a bit different from what you might be used to.

Take each step and stage as it comes and do it in a methodical manner so you always feel like you are achieving something every day. It is easy to get overwhelmed and confused and achieve nothing, but even easier to take things slowly and achieve everything.

15) I am very overweight – will this still work for me?
Yes indeed. In fact, the biggest success stories have been from those who had a significant amount to lose. It's a myth that those who have a lot of weight to come off are lazy etc. So often there is an element of low self-esteem attached, purely from dealing with society and its attitude to anyone 'different'.

So, when the mind set changes from what you don't want to do, to what you DO want, this has a dramatic effect on metabolism, state of mind, momentum and can have some quite exciting and dramatic effects. Anyone who feels they have a long way to go is always welcome to contact me for additional support.

16) Do I need to exercise as you mention in the book?
To be honest, for the best results, yes. Remember to read the section carefully though, as so many people advise methods which will slow down your metabolic rate rather than boost it, especially if you have an over-sensitive metabolism. It doesn't have to be radical or time consuming, you

just fit it in where you need to.

17) What is my ideal weight?
Your ideal weight is the size and shape you wish to be. When do you feel the best? When you are out in public and the shape you want to be, when you are feeling attractive and wonderful, or when you stand on the scales?

Other Titles From Mirage Publishing

A Prescription from The Love Doctor: How to find Love in 7 Easy Steps - Dr Joanne 'The Love Doctor' Coyle
Burnt: One Man's Inspiring Story of Survival - Ian Colquhoun
Cosmic Ordering Guide - Stephen Richards
Cosmic Ordering Connection - Stephen Richards
Cosmic Ordering: Chakra Clearing - Stephen Richards
Cosmic Ordering: Oracle Healing Cards – Stephen Richards
Cosmic Ordering: Oracle Wish Cards – Stephen Richards & Karen Whitelaw Smith
Cosmic Ordering: Rapid Chakra Clearing – Stephen Richards
Internet Dating King's Diaries: Life, Dating and Love – Clive Worth
Life Without Lottie: How I Coped (or didn't) During my Daughter's Gap Year - Fiona Fridd
Mrs Darley's Pagan Whispers: A Celebration of Pagan Festivals, Sacred Days, Spirituality and Traditions of the Year – Carole Carlton
Past Life Tourism - Barbara Ford-Hammond
Psychic Salon - Barbara Ford-Hammond
The Butterfly Experience: Inspiration For Change - Karen Whitelaw Smith
The Hell of Allegiance: My Living Nightmare of being Gang Raped and Held for Ten days by the British Army – Charmaine Maeer with Stephen Richards
The Real Office: An Uncharacteristic Gesture of Magnanimity by Management Supremo Hilary Wilson-Savage - Hilary Wilson-Savage
The Tumbler: Kassa (Košice) – Auschwitz – Sweden - Israel - Azriel Feuerstein

Mirage Publishing Website:
www.miragepublishing.com

Submissions of Mind, Body & Spirit manuscripts welcomed from new authors.